HEADACHE HELP

HEADACHE HELP

A COMPLETE GUIDE TO UNDERSTANDING HEADACHES AND THE MEDICINES THAT RELIEVE THEM

LAWRENCE ROBBINS, M.D., AND SUSAN S. LANG

Houghton Mifflin Company

BOSTON   NEW YORK

Library of Congress Cataloging-in-Publication Data

Robbins, Lawrence D.
Headache help : a complete guide to understanding headaches
and the medicines that relieve them / Lawrence Robbins and
Susan S. Lang
p.   cm.
Includes bibliographical references and index.
ISBN 0-395-70751-X
1. Headache — Popular works.   I. Lang, Susan S.   II. Title.
RB 128.R628   1995
616.8'491—dc20   94-43494
CIP

Book design by Anne Chalmers

Printed in the United States of America

QUM 10 9 8 7 6 5 4 3 2

The information presented in case histories and stories in *Headache Help* is medically accurate. However, all names, places, and identifying characteristics have
been changed to protect privacy. Some case histories contain elements from more
than one patient. Any resemblance to persons living or dead is coincidental.

Before you start the regimens presented in this book, consult your own physician
to make sure that they are suitable for you. None of the information here is in-
tended to substitute for medical advice. If you have any problems or questions related to your health and fitness, you should direct them to your physician.

For my family
and those suffering
the burden of head pain

— L.D.R.

For Solon J. Lang

— S.S.L.

THE GRIEF OF THE HEAD
IS THE GRIEF OF GRIEFS.

— James Howell,
English Proverbs, 1659

CONTENTS

· · · · · ·

~~~~~

PREFACE

· · · · · ·

~~~~~

HEADACHE is an extremely common problem that affects tens of millions of people in the United States. As a headache specialist who suffers from migraines and daily headaches myself, I know firsthand the burden that headaches add to one's life.

In the past ten years, there has been a virtual revolution in the understanding and treatment of headaches. Yet headaches remain largely misunderstood by many physicians and patients alike and, in general, remain a poorly treated condition. Like asthma, shock, epilepsy, and many other medical problems once thought to be caused by stress or emotions, headache is a legitimate physiological condition, not a psychological one. People who get headaches do not bring them on themselves but rather have different levels of the brain chemical serotonin and a much greater reactivity of blood vessels about the head than others.

Despite tremendous strides in headache management, enormous amounts of time and money are wasted on useless diagnostic tests and treatments. As a result, headache sufferers, who have been unfairly blamed for their illness for far too long, become angry and frustrated, and many simply give up the search for effective headache therapy.

Many of the books currently available on headaches emphasize nonmedication techniques, which can be very useful but often only up to a point. These books give precious little information about the vast array of effective medications now available. Headache sufferers want to know more about their medications, and they should. Susan Lang and I felt there was a need for a book about the actions and side effects of the drugs that readers may take and the trial and error that is sometimes necessary to find the right medication at the right dose.

That's why this book places a strong emphasis on drug therapy. Nonmedication techniques are important, and *Headache Help* explores them fully. But for those who suffer severe headaches, they tend to fall short and medication becomes the primary key to treatment. Our aim is to provide as much reference material as possible so that lay readers can be better informed.

Headache sufferers should be commended for fighting through life with head pain. We hope the burgeoning knowledge about headaches will lead to more compassion for their suffering. With our new understanding of headaches as a physical problem, we can help the vast majority of patients tremendously with current therapies. If you or a loved one suffers from head pain, you should know all about the options; hence, we give you this book.

A caveat: Although we discuss many medications and treatments for headaches, this information is not meant to be prescriptive, suggestive, or a substitute for the medical advice of a physician. Only your doctor, who understands your particular situation, can make well-informed decisions about your treatment plan. Similarly, although we offer lists of common or first-line medication choices, there are always exceptions and your doctor is best equipped to make this judgment.

Our intent is to provide information and education. In most cases, we could present only the common uses and side effects of medications. When you get a prescription, we still recommend that you ask your doctor or your pharmacist for details about possible side effects. *Physicians' Desk Reference* or the package insert also lists contraindications.

—Lawrence Robbins, M.D.
Northbrook, Illinois

～～～～～

SOME OF MY VIVID childhood memories are of my father's migraines. On bad days, he would retreat into his study and the house became dark and gloomy. Although we four children tried to remember to stay quiet, we often forgot and my mother would harshly scold us and banish us from the upstairs rooms. When would Daddy feel better and life resume its normal quality? Why did he have to get these things called migraines and disrupt our lives?

Since those days, my dad has "outgrown" his horrendous headaches, and we've emerged from the dark ages of headache treatments. But even the best treatments are useless if they are not sought out or adhered to. Information is empowering and is one of our most effective tools in our quest for better health and well-being. As a medical writer, my goal is to provide you with information so that you are not the passive recipient of a doctor's care, but an active, well-informed consumer.

I hope our use of gender pronouns will not offend anyone. Although many physicians are female, we have used masculine pronouns in most places to keep the language of the book simple.

Finally, to address those who may criticize Lawrence Robbins and me for focusing so heavily on medications: We do not minimize the power of mind-body techniques or of more natural therapies. Rather, we believe you should be fully informed of the full range of options. Only then can you properly weigh the risks and benefits of each potential therapy and weave your way through the maze of alternatives.

You deserve a pain-free life. We hope this book will help you achieve it.

—Susan S. Lang
Ithaca, New York

HEADACHE HELP

. . . .
〰〰〰〰〰

1

UNDERSTANDING
THE MODERN APPROACH

IF YOU'RE READING THIS BOOK, chances are you know the misery of headaches all too well. One moment life is normal, but the next your temples begin to ache and your forehead throbs. Soon your head is your worst enemy. The pounding, splitting pain of the headache overwhelms all else.

Contrary to what most people believe, you don't have to put up with it. If you get headaches frequently, don't despair; you can gain more control over them than you probably ever thought possible. Unfortunately, far too many people accept headaches as a fact of life. This attitude cheats you and your loved ones. Although headaches can't necessarily be cured, they can be controlled with certain lifestyle changes and, if needed, the wise and judicious use of modern medications.

Don't let headaches disrupt and complicate your life anymore. Take a stand. Learn what you can do to help yourself and your doctor to minimize the pain, agony, and frustration of headaches.

THE BAD NEWS

If you are one of the 45 to 50 million Americans who battle chronic headaches, you're probably not only miserable from the pain but guilty, depressed, and frustrated about missing work, disappointing loved ones, and giving up many of life's joys. You may fear that others view you as a malingerer, that your illness may jeopardize your job and future, and that maybe you are "crazy" and making yourself sick.

The truth is, headaches are a real physical illness and perhaps the most common medical condition plaguing human beings. They not only extort an exceedingly high price from individuals, but also from society. They are to blame for more than 157 million lost workdays a year in the United States at a price tag of some $50 billion in healthcare costs — including some 10 million office visits — and absenteeism.

The costly toll of headaches could be greatly reduced by better understanding how your lifestyle contributes to your headache pattern; how nondrug strategies, such as relaxation techniques, biofeedback, diet changes, and exercise, can make a significant impact; and how to use the right medication, chosen from a large and powerful arsenal. All you need is information, a willingness and commitment to try nondrug strategies, and in many cases, a trial-and-error approach to medication.

THE GOOD NEWS THAT FEW USE

Ironically, while a revolution has occurred in the headache field over the past ten years, most people who get headaches have failed to reap the benefits. Medical researchers understand the mechanisms of headache better than ever before. They have unlocked the mystery of how certain triggers set off headaches and how lifestyle changes can ward off many attacks. They have developed exquisitely specific headache medications that can quickly relieve or abort a potentially devastating headache. And for people who get frequent headaches, medical researchers now know how to stabilize someone with low doses of certain medications to make him less sensitive to headache triggers, thereby preventing many headaches from recurring.

Yet, tragically, although headache doctors now have the medical know-how to help more than 90 percent of headache sufferers, more than 70 percent of sufferers never even consult a doctor about their headaches.

WHY HEADACHES FAIL TO GET TREATED

Despite all the recent medical advances, many headache consumers passively endure the agony. Why? Because they mistakenly believe that little can be done to help them. Even worse, some people unwittingly aggravate their headaches by taking too many over-the-counter and prescription pain relievers and loading up on caffeine. Or they fail to give proven nondrug strategies, such as relaxation and other stress-reduction methods and exercise, a concerted try.

Others fail to seek medical help that could provide drugs that might change their lives. Of those who do consult doctors, many become quickly discouraged. Sometimes doctors are unaware of the latest treatments. Other times, however, consumers are given appropriate advice but are too suspicious of what may sound like a newfangled advance. Some patients think the doctor is fishing in the dark when the first medication doesn't work and a completely different one is prescribed. Although the doctor is following a very clear and reasonable strategy that often requires trial and error, the patient who is unaware of his rationale may become confused.

Still others may start a prescription medication but soon quit it and they frequently never follow up with the doctor if it doesn't work or causes too many side effects. Some headache sufferers so fear the shift from a medication-free life to one suddenly cluttered with strange pills that they refuse to take their medicines consistently or correctly.

Instead, people spend billions of dollars trying all kinds of treatments on their own. Although some of these nondrug, natural approaches, especially relaxation and coping techniques, diet, and exercise, can and do prevent some headaches, many people still needlessly suffer because they either do not effectively institute the lifestyle changes required or because their headaches also require medication for relief.

HEADACHES ARE A REAL PHYSICAL ILLNESS

Before we get into the nitty-gritty details of treatment strategies, we need to get something straight: headaches are not psychological illnesses simply induced by stress but are genuine medical illnesses as legitimate as ulcers, diabetes, or heart disease. Stress may contribute to the muscle tension in the head or changes in the brain's blood vessels that cause pain, but researchers now know that headache mechanisms involve involuntary biochemical changes in the brain.

If you get chronic headaches, chances are you suffer from the bad luck of being born with a slightly different brain chemistry than most people, a sort of short circuit. In fact, the gene location for migraine is very close to being identified and may contribute to the irregular brain chemistry. Researchers strongly suspect that this different brain chemistry makes you more prone to painful dilated blood vessels in your head, and to the uncontrollable firing of the nerve cells in the transmission of pain signals. In other words, your brain chemistry makes you more likely to get headaches.

WHAT CAUSES AND TRIGGERS HEADACHES?

Although scientists still don't know the exact causes of headaches, many are convinced that the primary culprits are imbalances in the brain's chemicals and nerve pathways. The latest and most widely accepted theory is that the majority of headaches — namely tension headaches and migraines, which are thought to be on opposite ends of a spectrum — are caused by the depletion of the chemical serotonin, a neurotransmitter (brain protein) that is involved in communication among nerve cells in the brain.

Serotonin plays an important role in regulating the diameter of blood vessels, that is, in constricting and expanding them, and, as we've said, it is the dilation of blood vessels which causes pain. Serotonin also stifles pain signals between nerve cells and influences sleep, anxiety, and mood (and is key to depression). Stress and other environmental factors are thought to influence levels of serotonin in the brain.

In normal cases, nerves that surround the blood vessels in the brain's protective covering, the meninges, release normal levels of neurotransmitters like serotonin and no pain occurs. In headache cases, however, certain factors, such as stress or a particular food, trigger a chain of events in people born with troublesome serotonin regulation. Researchers think that first a wave of electrical activity spreads over the brain. Then the level of serotonin surges and blood vessels around the brain constrict. Consequently, as the serotonin seeps into surrounding tissues, levels of the neurotransmitter fall in the brain. This decrease in serotonin causes the blood vessels to become inflamed and swollen, irritating surrounding nerves and perhaps the trigeminal nerve, a large and complicated nerve that extends to the blood vessels around the brain and into the face. The inflammation of the blood vessels and the irritation of nerves cause pain.

The serotonin pathways that play a vital role in migraines and probably tension headaches are the same pathways that influence depression, anxiety, and insomnia. Researchers have recently discovered that people with migraines in particular have a higher risk of depression, anxiety, and mild insomnia. While frequent headaches may cause a person to feel depressed or anxious, studies show that the increased risk of these conditions is independent of the headaches themselves. Migraine sufferers do, however, have much higher rates of panic attacks and moderately higher levels of chronic mild anxiety and nervousness (especially when the headaches are out of control), as well as more depression than people in the general population. Depression may aggravate preexisting headaches, but it does not cause headaches.

Serotonin attaches only to certain receptors in the brain, and different receptors may be associated with different conditions, such as headache, depression, and anxiety. Medications that fit on the serotonin receptors, and thereby mimic serotonin (such as sumatriptan), or influence serotonin levels (such as DHE, dihydroergotamine, and antidepressants) can help prevent and relieve both migraine and tension headaches. Other kinds of medications may help by either blocking the pain message, by constricting the swollen and inflamed blood vessels, or by stabilizing the blood vessels so they don't swell. Interestingly, many medications used for years because of their influence on blood vessels recently have been found to influence serotonin levels as well.

The muscles in the head may also contribute to headache pain by tightening up. But this occurrence is now believed to be the result of the headache mechanism rather than a cause of it. Nevertheless, once the muscles contract, they may contribute to the pain by releasing a toxic by-product, lactic acid, and reducing the amount of blood and oxygen that can get into the muscles.

Of course, not everyone gets chronic headaches. But if you are prone to headaches, probably because of some genetic or biochemical predisposition, serotonin imbalances probably occur more easily in you than in other people due to certain environmental, chemical, physical, and psychological factors. These triggers, which differ among individuals, include certain foods like chocolate and alcohol, bright lights, hunger, a changing sleep schedule, a hormonal shift, or psychological conditions like stress, anxiety, and depression. Sometimes even high altitudes, orgasm, and exercise may trigger headaches. Again, these factors aren't the causes of headaches; rather, they aggravate the biological condition that promotes the headaches. But by identifying which factors trigger your headaches and how to avoid them, you can learn how to relieve and prevent them.

TOO MUCH OF A GOOD THING: REBOUND HEADACHES

Ironically, people who suffer from chronic headaches all too often unwittingly make themselves sicker by overusing headache medications in their quest for relief. Too much caffeine — more than what is in three or four cups of coffee a day or in a more-than-twice-weekly dose of some pain relievers or decongestants — can seriously aggravate headaches. Even just two aspirin and some caffeine every day can turn occasional headaches into a chronic and severe headache problem while also making you less sensitive to many medications that might have helped you relieve or prevent the headache in the first place. Some 50 to 80 percent of all headache sufferers unknowingly fall victim to rebound headaches.

Unfortunately, it's all too easy to get caught in the rebound headache trap. Here's a typical scenario: You get a headache and find that a lot of caffeine or an analgesic, such as aspirin, ibuprofen (Motrin, Nuprin, Advil), acetaminophen (Tylenol), or a prescription vasoconstrictor (ergotamine) relieves it. Because it is so effective, you start taking it more freely. As your headaches escalate, so does your use of the caffeine or analgesic. As a result of the overuse, however, the substance becomes increasingly less effective — either because your blood vessels become somewhat immune to the substance or because the substance interferes with your body's ability to produce endorphins (natural morphine-like substances produced by your brain). As you become less sensitive to the caffeine or medication, you may try taking even more or try a new medication. The final result is that you end up with more frequent and severe headaches, and if you cut down, you still get headaches. In the case of caffeine, you may get weekend headaches if you drink far less coffee on Saturdays and Sundays than during the week.

So the very medications that can be most useful for headache relief can become your worst enemy. This syndrome is so common that some experts describe rebound headaches as an "unrecognized epidemic" in this country. In some cases, people must be hospitalized to go through the uncomfortable withdrawal process, which includes severe headaches. Ironically, withdrawal is all that is required in many cases to achieve significant relief from a chronic headache problem.

Because rebound headaches are so common among all kinds of headache sufferers, learning how to balance your use of medications and caffeine can determine whether these substances will be among your best friends or ugly enemies.

HOW DOCTORS TREAT HEADACHES

If you suffer frequently from chronic headaches, your first goal is to do everything you can to avoid them by becoming well informed about foods and substances that may trigger them and how relaxation and coping skills, exercise, caffeine, and over-the-counter (OTC) pain relievers may help. If these approaches don't work, you should consult a doctor and ask about stronger, abortive medication to relieve a headache. Commonly, abortive medications, such as Midrin or Norgesic Forte, are used to prevent a mild or moderate headache from becoming severe. Other abortive medications, such as sumatriptan (Imitrex), can relieve a headache that has already become severe.

If you suffer from moderate to severe headaches more than three times a month and these episodes are severe enough to interfere with your family, job, or social life, then your doctor may recommend a preventive medication as well. Such drugs are not always completely effective, but they can minimize the frequency of headaches and the disruption to your life.

Many people don't want to take preventive medication because it means daily pill-popping. However, if you get frequent severe headaches that seriously impair your ability to get on with life's routines, your doctor may suggest switching from abortive medication each time you get a headache to preventive medication. Preventives are not only more benign than the abortives, but you end up taking less medication with preventives than if you just chase the pain with abortives. Also, abortive medications tend to be more addicting and have more side effects than preventive medication. We'll discuss guidelines for these strategies in subsequent chapters.

You must realize that trying a medication regimen is not a permanent decision with lasting side effects. Medications may be used as temporary stopgaps to control a period when the headaches seem particularly overwhelming. After a spell, when the brain's misfirings seem to quiet down, you may go for months using only lifestyle techniques to prevent attacks. Then, for unpredictable reasons, if your biological mechanisms fire up again and set off another bad run of headaches, you may need abortive or preventive medications again for some time.

This is why becoming familiar with a headache doctor's medical approach is so important. By understanding the basic strategy — abortive versus preventive, as well as the options, risks, and benefits of each — you can make appropriate, well-informed decisions with your doctor. Then, using a rational, trial-and-error approach, you can decide together how to proceed if a medication is ineffective or has too many side effects.

TRIAL AND ERROR

Although lifestyle strategies that involve diet, exercise, relaxation, and the moderate use of caffeine and over-the-counter pain relievers (see Chapter 2) can help prevent headaches, when they fail to work as reliably as you'd hoped, prescription medications are the next resort. Only they can compensate for the differences in the brain chemistry or blood vessel changes that cause pain.

However, treating headaches is both an art and a science, and often the first try doesn't work. Each person is different: your headaches may be triggered by factors very different from someone else's and your response to medications is also unique. You need to work patiently in partnership with your doctor, who may need to experiment with doses, monitor you for side effects, and recommend several changes in medication before getting the right balance. Even after you find the right medication and correct doses, over time the medication may become less effective and your doctor may have to experiment again. At times this trial-and-error process may be frustrating, but try not to give up: The hope for a higher quality of life with fewer headaches should make up for the setbacks and stumbling blocks you may encounter along the way.

NONHEADACHE MEDICINES

You may wonder why your doctor would prescribe an antidepressant, anticonvulsant, or perhaps a medication used for high blood pressure or heart disease for your headaches. This approach isn't as odd as you may think. Certain medications commonly used to treat headaches are not always specifically approved or indicated by the Food and Drug Administration for this purpose. However, this practice is common. Medications often have several, sometimes a dozen, different effects. When drug companies develop and test a new medication — say, a drug with antidepressant, analgesic, sedative, and anti-seizure effects — they focus on whatever property they think will be most marketable or profitable. In this case, they may focus their very costly research efforts on the drug's ability to prevent seizures. Once the drug is approved by the Food and Drug Administration as a safe and effective anticonvulsant, doctors may then decide to use it for an altogether different purpose.

Since swollen blood vessels are a primary cause of head pain, many medications used for headaches have a beneficial effect on blood vessels. The medications either influence serotonin, which in turn helps control blood vessel constriction and dilation; constrict swollen blood vessels directly; or help prevent blood vessels from swelling in the first place. Other medications, however, such as narcotics, help headaches by dulling the pain signal to the brain.

WHAT KIND OF HEADACHE DO YOU GET?

One of the first steps to understanding your head pain is to identify what kinds of headaches you get. Although there are about a dozen major types and more than sixty subtypes of headaches, the vast majority are either migraines or tension headaches, which most people will get from time to time, and to a lesser extent, cluster headaches. Many headaches that are believed to be common, such as sinus headaches and allergy headaches, are, in fact, quite uncommon. Many other types of headaches are, actually very rare and caused by serious disorders, such as brain tumors or meningitis, and can be identified by certain high-risk factors. See Chapter 2, "Symptoms to Take Seriously."

MIGRAINES

Migraines may afflict up to twenty-five million Americans, two-thirds of them women, many of whom get menstrual headaches as well. Migraines, which are usually inherited, are characterized by throbbing or aching pain, usually on one side of the head, and are often coupled with nausea and sometimes vomiting, visual disturbances, or dizziness. Numbness in an arm or area of the face may also occur. Some sufferers get so-called classic migraines with aura — they see colors, shimmering lights, or experience other kinds of visual changes. Without auras, the headaches are called common migraines.

TENSION OR MUSCLE-CONTRACTION HEADACHES

More than three-quarters of all headaches are tension headaches, previously called muscle-contraction headaches. Typically, as muscles tighten in your head and neck and blood vessels in your head expand, you feel a throbbing forehead pain, a dull pain on both sides of the head, or a sensation that your head is being squeezed, tightened, or pressed, as if in a vise. Although the name is "tension headache," stress and tension are not the major precipitating factors. Although we all get these headaches occasionally, some poor souls get them often, sometimes every day or every other day. When these headaches are chronic, they are, like migraines, often the result of a genetically inherited, predetermined condition. Although the pain may stem partly from the muscles over the head contracting, researchers now believe that the root causes of tension headaches

CHARACTERISTICS OF THE MOST COMMON HEADACHES

Type of Headache	Onset	Pain	Who Gets Them	Pattern	Duration	Other Symptoms
MIGRAINES	Usually in childhood or by late twenties	Moderate to severe; usually one-sided; near an eye; pulsating or throbbing	70% are women	Several a month (from several weekly to several yearly)	Average: 4–8 hours; may last days	Visual disturbances; nausea/vomiting; dizziness; sensitivity to light and noise
TENSION	Any time	Mild to moderate; like a band or vise; across temples or head; usually not debilitating	Slightly more women than men	No periodocity	No clear beginning or end	Tightness in neck and shoulders
CLUSTER	In mid-life (between ages 20 and 45)	Excruciating; one-sided; sharp, like a knife	80% are men	Occur in clusters of time, usually weeks to months once or twice a year	½ hour –1 hour	Flushed face; teary eye; stuffed or runny nose

are the same as those of migraines: serotonin imbalances and blood vessel changes. When chronic, these headaches often need something stronger than over-the-counter pain relievers. And as with migraines, the use of OTC pain relievers can backfire and make these headaches worse.

CLUSTER HEADACHES

Afflicting about 1 out of 250 men and 1 out of 1,000 women, these agonizing headaches are among the most severe pains known to humankind. Their excruciating, debilitating pain, sometimes described as a red-hot iron being twisted around or through an eye or a temple, may last from fifteen minutes to three hours, sometimes longer. They're called cluster headaches because they occur in waves, usually lasting several weeks to several months, once or twice a year. Symptoms that commonly occur with clusters include a runny or stuffed nose, a teary or red eye, or a drooping eyelid on the same side as the pain.

LESS COMMON HEADACHES

POST-TRAUMATIC HEADACHES are the result of injuries from an accident (especially a car accident) in which the head or neck is involved.

SINUS HEADACHES are linked to colds, a runny nose, or hay fever and are not as common as you think. Most people who believe (or have been told) that they have sinus headaches (and get relief from decongestants) actually experience tension headaches or migraines (for which the decongestants may help because they contain caffeine) that are causing pain in the sinus region.

TMJ HEADACHES are also much rarer than most people believe. Although TMJ (temporomandibular jaw syndrome) causes face pain and sometimes a headache, most chronic headaches in TMJ sufferers are actually migraines or chronic tension headaches. The TMJ may aggravate the preexisting migraine or tension headache problem.

EXERCISE AND SEXUAL HEADACHES may occur at any age, especially after exercise such as weightlifting, soccer in which the head is used, aerobics, jogging, diving, and sex. These headaches are usually benign (although they can be serious in rare cases) and often last only about twenty minutes, but sometimes as long as a day. Consult a physician if you experience exercise or sexual headaches.

ALLERGY HEADACHES are, in fact, rare. Most so-called allergy headaches are reactions, but not true allergic responses, to certain chemicals in foods that commonly trigger headaches. A mild headache may occur due to nasal or sinus congestion because of the allergies.

And as you'll see in later chapters, other factors, such as eyestrain, caffeine withdrawal, ear infections, an overactive thyroid, and dental problems can also cause headaches. Serious problems are rare, but you should rule them out by consulting a physician.

HOW HEADACHES AFFECT COUPLES AND FAMILIES

Although headaches are a legitimate illness, many families and coworkers tend to be less sympathetic to headaches than to other sicknesses. Yet the effects of headaches may ripple through a family profoundly. When you get headaches, you may fail to fulfill your commitments as a spouse or parent because of the pain. When you suffer, your mate suffers too, driving you to the emergency room, making midnight dashes to the pharmacy, calling the doctor at all hours, preparing ice packs in the middle of the night, breaking plans, feeling emotionally and physically drained, bearing the burden of additional medical bills, coping with added child care and home responsibilities, trying to stay sympathetic to your moodiness during and after the headache, working with you regarding drug overuse or abuse, and so on, all due to your severe head pain.

You may have feelings of guilt, shame, anger, isolation, and inadequacy. Although you certainly are suffering, try to understand how your illness affects those around you as well. Chronic headaches are often a source of strife between partners. Some mates don't understand that the pain is the result of an inherited physical illness that is no more psychological than any other illness. Others fear that their partners take too much headache medication; although this may sometimes be true, it often is not. Yet it may appear to be a problem to a partner who doesn't understand why there are so many pill bottles in the medicine chest. Many headache sufferers need an array of choices — not only a pain reliever and perhaps a preventive medication, but also choices among these medications, depending on whether the headache strikes at night or during the day and whether they need to go to work or not. They may also need an antinausea medication. In addition, they may get new prescriptions when the current medication isn't strong enough but they keep the old prescription in case the new medication has too many side effects. The overwhelming majority of headache sufferers take medication simply for pain and nausea and do not abuse these medications for recreational use (although many do overuse them for pain).

Although headache sufferers are no more or less prone to addiction than others and simply wish to relieve their pain, family members may not understand and raise issues concerning medications and failed expectations. Your partner may need to suppress his own needs at times to care for you. This is tough when the headaches are chronic. Both of you need to try to understand each other's lot.

QUALITY OF LIFE

Medical researchers have made great strides in treating headache. A wide array of relaxation techniques and medications are available. The choices are wide, and finding the right one may take some time and trial and error. With proper treatment, you can learn how to gain control over your life, enjoy relief and a restored high quality of life. We offer rational and reasonable strategies for a range of headache situations.

The road isn't straight, and often what seemed to be the right path becomes a dead end. You may have to backtrack, but it's worth it. After all, your life — and whether head pain will interfere with it or not — is what's at stake.

2

....

HELPING YOURSELF

IF YOU GET frequent or severe headaches, you need to consult a physician. Nevertheless, you may want to know how to help yourself both with short-term techniques to get rid of a headache and long-term techniques to prevent future headaches.

Chances are, these self-help strategies won't always work, but if they can ward off some of your headaches so much the better. Before you consider self-help methods, however, you should understand that there may be something more serious going on than just a headache. If the following symptoms occur, consult a doctor as soon as possible.

SYMPTOMS TO TAKE SERIOUSLY

- The headaches get progressively worse over days or weeks.
- The headaches have started suddenly; you've never had them before (especially important if you're over fifty).
- The headache comes on suddenly after coughing, straining, or exertion, which has never happened before.
- You experience changes in memory, personality, behavior, or level of consciousness (that is, you become confused).
- You experience changes in vision or in your ability to walk, general weakness, numbness, or loss of senses.

- You have a stiff neck with a fever or a rash, or you experience a seizure.
- You have an unexplained fever or breathing problems, as well as the headache.
- There is a sudden or dramatic change in the severity of your headaches. If you get a very sudden and excruciating headache unlike any you've ever had, consult a doctor immediately.
- You get a headache after a head injury or accident, or after a sore throat or respiratory infection.
- You have a constant headache with no relief.

Assuming your physician rules out the possibility of a serious illness, here is a summary of the general guidelines for self-help methods to control headaches, which we'll examine in detail in this chapter.

HOW TO GET RID OF A HEADACHE: PRACTICAL STRATEGIES

- Practice a relaxation exercise.
- Drink something with caffeine, such as cola or coffee, or take a caffeine tablet.
- Try aspirin, ibuprofen (Motrin, Advil), or acetaminophen but not more than twice a week. The sooner you take it, the better.
- Apply reusable ice packs to the painful area.
- Try to sleep in a dark and quiet room.

RELAXATION AND DEEP-BREATHING EXERCISES

Far too many people discount the value of relaxation and deep-breathing exercises. Although considered totally unconventional just twenty years ago, these techniques have been successful in the East for centuries and Western scientists have recently become more convinced of their powerful and beneficial physiological and psychological effects. They are now more widely accepted than ever before and are used in hospitals and clinics throughout the country as effective, legitimate, no-risk techniques.

If your pain is still somewhat mild, before reaching for a pill try just twenty to thirty seconds of a relaxation exercise, especially deep breathing and imagery techniques.

Relaxation in this context does not mean putting your feet up and reading the newspaper or watching TV. Rather, it is a technique to induce deep physical relaxation that reduces the body's response to stress by quieting both the mind and body. Physiologically, it can relieve pain by lowering your blood pressure, breathing rate, and pulse; reducing muscle tension and muscle spasms in your head and neck; increasing blood flow; and even stimulating brain waves associated with peace and tranquillity. Psychologically, these techniques help reduce distress, anxiety, and depression and promote a greater sense of calm, all of which can reduce pain.

Deep relaxation can also help change your perception and experience of pain and your response to it. By learning how to reduce the ill effects of stress, including its contribution to headaches, you gain a greater sense of control and mastery over your response to the stress. That control may also boost your hope and optimism and make you less conscious of your pain.

Many studies have shown the beneficial effects of relaxation and deep-breathing exercises. For example, during painful procedures, such as bone marrow transplants, when people practice relaxation methods, they have significantly lower pain ratings and pulse rates than when they take a tranquilizer or are distracted by videos. At Duke University, it has been shown that relaxation can help relieve lower back pain. And at the State University of New York at Albany, relaxation has been shown to help directly with chronic headache. Nausea and vomiting, which sometimes occur with migraines and headache medications, can also be significantly relieved with relaxation methods.

Unfortunately, although more doctors are now convinced of relaxation's beneficial effects, many people are unwilling to learn them or to stick with these methods for very long. Some people resent being asked to try these techniques, believing they are mere mental tricks that minimize the legitimacy of their pain and suffering. Others feel silly or have no faith that they can help.

Yet if you acknowledge that pain escalates when you're upset, then you can understand how the opposite can be true: pain can be soothed when you're more relaxed. Also, because these techniques are safe, noninvasive, and have no risk of side effects, trying them can't hurt.

A few cautionary notes, however, are in order. These exercises are skills and as such they must be learned, practiced, and mastered. They cannot be adopted passively. They will be most effective for mild pain and can often avert the need to take an over-the-counter analgesic. Don't be discouraged if they don't seem to help on the first try. It may take up to two weeks to feel comfortable with these skills and to produce a beneficial effect.

PROMOTING RELAXATION

Various methods are commonly used to achieve deep relaxation, or what Dr. Herbert Benson has called the "relaxation response." These techniques include breathing exercises, physical exercise, visualization, autogenic training, progressive muscle relaxation, and biofeedback. Different people prefer different techniques. Use the one that helps you most easily achieve a sense of inner calm and peace. If you are able and willing to use your imagination with confidence, you will achieve the best results.

At first, try these techniques in a quiet location, sitting or lying down in a comfortable position with your eyes closed. Listening to soothing background music may further help promote a sense of calm. Once you become used to these exercises, you may be able to do some of them at work or even while driving (with your eyes open, of course).

CONTROLLED BREATHING OR MEDITATION Focus all your attention on your breathing for at least twenty to thirty seconds. Optimally, breathe deeply, slowly, and rhythmically, through your nose, deep in the back of the throat so you can actually hear your breathing. Hold the breaths for several seconds and exhale very slowly, completely emptying your lungs. Try tensing different muscles when you inhale and relax them when you exhale. Start with the toes and feet, and work your way up to your head. Some trainers suggest that upon exhaling you say a calming word or mantra to yourself (such as "relax," "peace," "beauty," or "love").

EXERCISE Any aerobic exercise, such as walking, biking, taking an exercise class, swimming, or playing tennis for at least thirty minutes, five times a week, can make a significant impact in preventing headaches. Regular aerobic exercise not only promotes the physiological relaxation response but boosts the production of endorphins (as does laughter and being in love), morphinelike chemicals that the brain produces. Endorphins give us a sense of well-being, raising our pain threshold as well as stimulating circulation, which bathes tissues in more oxygen and flushes out the body's toxins more quickly. Exercise may also be important in countering the effects of taking pain relievers frequently, as some researchers believe that frequent use of these medications may impair the brain's ability to produce endorphins. In addition to all its other benefits, exercise has also been shown to reduce stress, depression, and anxiety, which, in turn, can raise your pain threshold.

VISUALIZATION This technique can be added to the deep-breathing exercises. Visualization, also known as imagery, involves conjuring up a pleasant picture, imagining that you are in a beautiful garden, for instance, feeling soothed and relaxed. Visualization may also involve using your mind to imagine that physical changes are occurring. Pretend, for instance, that a magic wand is passing over your painful swollen blood vessels and causing them to constrict.

Many studies have found that there is more to these techniques than just taking your mind temporarily off the pain. By concentrating on pleasant scenes or magic wands that produce change, you can actually stimulate the same parts of the brain that are activated when you are experiencing the tranquil scene in reality, producing beneficial physiological changes that help promote relief for mild to moderate pain.

VISUALIZATION EXERCISE TO PROMOTE RELAXATION

Get as comfortable as possible and close your eyes.

You are on a tropical beach, and warm, soothing breezes are flowing over you. Imagine that you are floating dreamily on a raft in crystal-clear turquoise water. Feel the sun warming your body as the raft gently rocks up and down.

Imagine that the heat of the sun is warming your fingertips, your arms, your toes, your legs; it is bathing your painful forehead in its healing light.

Feel the bobbing motion and try to feel as weightless as possible.

Breathe slowly and deeply. Soon you are floating higher and higher, up to a large, beautiful cloud, drifting through the sky.

Imagine only calmness, warmth, and peace.

Other images to try are a crackling fireplace or a cool expanse of luxurious lawn.

Rather than focusing on relaxation only, you can also use a similar exercise directly on a painful area:

VISUALIZATION EXERCISE FOR PAIN RELIEF

Breathe slowly, deeply, and evenly. In your mind's eye, imagine that a magic wand is coursing over your head, bathing it in healing energy. As you inhale, pretend that you are bringing in warm goodness and healing energy. Hold your incoming breath as long as possible, and during that time imagine that you are squeezing and tightening the painful blood vessels in your head. Then imagine that the blood is flowing from your head, where all this pressure is, to your fingertips. As you exhale, imagine that pain, tension, and poisons are flushed out with your breaths.

AUTOGENIC TRAINING This technique is relatively simple. Repeat self-affirming statements involving warmth, heaviness, and calmness. By repeating the statements over and over, you lull yourself into a sense of calm and tranquillity, thereby promoting the relaxation response. At the same time, you may be able to warm your hands and feet if they tend to get cold (as they often do with migraines).

EXERCISE FOR AUTOGENIC TRAINING

In a dark room, close your eyes and get as comfortable as possible.

Repeat each phrase four or five times. For example: "My forehead feels heavy and warm, very heavy and warm. My forehead is getting even heavier and warmer.

> *My forehead is sinking, sinking down into the pillow."*
> *As you repeat your phrases, conjure up an image, as you would in the visualization exercise, of a scene that brings warmth and pleasure. Repeat the phrases, each time substituting a different part of the head for "forehead" (eyes, sinuses, temples, top of the head, and so on), all the while breathing deeply and slowly. Your goal is to put your mind and body into a relaxed trance.*

PROGRESSIVE RELAXATION TRAINING   PRT involves tensing a part of the body, such as the hands or legs, for ten seconds, then releasing it from the tension. You squeeze each body part separately and sequentially, including every part you can think of, such as your forehead, eyes, and mouth, right down to your arms and fingers, feet and toes. After ten or fifteen minutes, you tense up the whole body and then allow it to go limp, releasing all tension.

Since many of us don't realize just how tense we really are and where we hold the tension in our bodies (neck or shoulder tension often contributes to headaches), PRT can help you identify the location of the tension and force you to relax. Several studies have shown that PRT can significantly reduce the severity and duration of nausea for cancer patients before chemotherapy (anticipatory nausea) and thus it may be useful to combat nausea linked to headaches.

SELF-HYPNOSIS   Self-hypnosis integrates the techniques already described, namely deep breathing, visualization, and progressive relaxation training, to achieve the same deep relaxation response and imagery to transform the pain sensations. The goal is to achieve a floating or drifting feeling, similar to your state just before falling asleep.

EXERCISE FOR SELF-HYPNOSIS

Sit or lie down in a comfortable position. Close your eyes.

Relax your body as much as possible. Release any tension held until you feel limp and loose.

Then focus on your toes. Are they feeling limp? They should feel heavy. Be sure to release all tension. Then move to your feet. Do they feel limp and heavy?

Move up your leg, letting tension go each step of the way. Keep moving through your body, concentrating on each part and releasing all the tension in it. Tell yourself you need to let go completely and relax.

Breathe evenly and deeply, trying to focus your mind on the rhythm of the breathing, on the sense of feeling sleepy and deeply relaxed. Your entire body will soon feel heavy, limp, and loose. When you're done, open your eyes, slowly sit up, and then stand.

BIOFEEDBACK   Biofeedback uses electronic equipment to monitor how successful you are with relaxation techniques to produce physiological changes. Biofeedback has been shown to help up to two-thirds of all headache sufferers who give it an earnest try. It is especially effective for teaching children and resistant adults that they can, in fact, exert some control over their body's response to stress.

By using painless electrodes on certain muscles and parts of the body, biofeedback electronically monitors body functions, such as breathing rate, blood circulation, heart rate, temperature, muscle tension, blood pressure, brain activity, and pulse. While being monitored, you practice the relaxation method of your choice and watch the instruments to see if you are actually producing physiological changes.

Temperature or thermal biofeedback can be very effective for migraines by helping you learn how to raise the temperature of your fingertips and achieve a relaxed state. The equipment lets you know how successful you are. Electromyographic bio-feedback, on the other hand, which electronically monitors muscle activity, can sometimes be particularly useful for tension headaches by helping you learn how to release muscle tension.

Most pain clinics and hospitals have biofeedback equipment; however, sessions may be costly. Once you learn how to produce those physiological changes reliably, you will no longer need the machine to check you. For more information and referrals, see Appendix A.

MASSAGE, WARM BATHS, HOT TUBS, AND YOGA Combined with controlled breathing, any of these relaxation techniques may help you release tension and is worth a try to relieve mild headache pain.

Many audiotapes, available through bookstores and health magazines, can lead you through such meditations and relaxation exercises. Although not for everyone, such tapes, with their soothing background music or white noise (the sound of a night forest, for example) may help you drift into a trance, far from your painful headache. Many people feel refreshed, relaxed, and calm after listening. You may find it more useful to make your own tapes, with music and imagery you prefer.

CAFFEINE

In addition to a few moments of a relaxation exercise, you can help ward off a brewing and still somewhat mild migraine or tension headache by drinking a few cups of caffeinated tea, coffee, or a soft drink, particularly if you don't consume a lot of caffeine on headache-free days. Caffeine may help because it constricts dilated blood vessels, which often cause the pain. Caffeine may also raise serotonin levels, according to some studies. Because it is moderately effective in warding off headaches, caffeine is an ingredient in many over-the-counter pain relievers.

The best strategy for using caffeine is either to avoid caffeine completely on headache-free days or to keep your consumption down to one or two cups a day. Then if you feel a headache beginning, have a nice strong cup or two of your favorite caffeinated drink. The beneficial effect should last several hours; if you feel the headache creeping back again, you can have another cup.

If you don't want to have a caffeine drink, try a caffeine tablet that you can buy at the pharmacy. The rule of thumb is to take about fifty milligrams every three or four hours, as needed. Try to limit caffeine to two hundred milligrams, or, at most, three hundred milligrams per day. Your limit will depend on your sleep patterns, whether you suffer from anxiety, and if you are sensitive to rebound headaches. To see how much caffeine is present in different foods and medications, consider the following table.

We can't stress enough that caffeine (and the pain relievers you'll read about in the next section) can also be one of your

CAFFEINE IN DRINKS, FOODS, AND MEDICATIONS

FOODS AND DRINKS	CAFFEINE
Brewed coffee	75–125 mg per cup (drip is stronger than percolated)
Instant coffee	40 mg, but sometimes up to 150 mg, per cup
Decaffeinated coffee	2–5 mg per cup
Tea	30–50 mg per cup
Soft drink	40 mg per cup

Chocolate	1–15 mg per oz
Cocoa	Up to 50 mg per cup
Caffeine tablet	100 mg
(No Doz, Tirend, and Vivarin; higher-strength tablets are available but not usually recommended.)	

MEDICATIONS	CAFFEINE
Excedrin Extra-Strength	65 mg per dose
Anacin	32 mg per dose
Vanquish	33 mg per dose
Bromo Seltzer, Cope, Midol	30–33 mg per dose

(Appendix B lists the caffeine content of most over-the-counter medications used for headache.)

worst enemies. If you drink more than two cups of coffee or tea daily during the week but not on weekends, you're likely to get headaches from caffeine withdrawal. These rebound headaches flare up when the effect of the caffeine wears off after your body has grown accustomed to it.

If you're now consuming a lot of caffeine regularly, try to taper it to only one or two cups a day. Then you'll be able to use the caffeine to your advantage.

To enhance the pain-relieving effect of caffeine, you may also want to take one of the over-the-counter pain relievers discussed in the following section.

OVER-THE-COUNTER PAIN RELIEVERS

When you've truly tried relaxation exercise and caffeine, to no avail, an over-the-counter pain reliever may be strong enough to help, especially if it is taken during the early stages of the headache. These pain relievers are combinations or single formulations of aspirin (or acetaminophen, Tylenol's main ingredient), with or without caffeine, and naproxen and ibuprofen, nonsteroidal anti-inflammatory drugs (NSAIDs). For the majority of people who get headaches, these medications are all they need.

But again, we must warn you about the risk of rebound headaches from taking these medications too often. Some people develop rebound headaches with as few as two or three of these pain relievers a day; others may not experience rebounds until they are consuming six or eight tablets a day. Nevertheless, it is important not to use these medications daily, but to restrict them to no more than twice a week. If you feel the need to use them more often, you should consult a doctor. Also, be sure not to mix more than one kind in the same day.

The best over-the-counter pain reliever for you will largely depend on your ability to tolerate the strongest ones. If nausea is a problem, you're well advised to avoid products with aspirin and the nonsteroidal anti-inflammatories. The medications in the following list appear in order of effectiveness, from most to least. Keep in mind that the stronger formulations are also more likely to cause side effects, particularly stomach or gastrointestinal irritation.

THE MOST USEFUL OVER-THE-COUNTER PAIN RELIEVERS FOR HEADACHES

1. EXCEDRIN EXTRA-STRENGTH OR COMPARABLE PRODUCTS (ANODYNOS, BC POWDER, BC TABLETS, BUFFETS II, COPE, DURADYNE, MIDOL, PRESALIN, S-A-C TABLETS, SALATIN, SALETO, SUPAC, TRIGESIC, TRI-PAIN, VANQUISH)

Excedrin Extra-Strength contains acetaminophen (250 mg), aspirin (250 mg), and more caffeine (65 mg) than Anacin, which usually makes it more effective but also more likely to lead to caffeine rebound headaches when medication is stopped.

TYPICAL DOSE: One or two tablets every three hours as needed. To prevent rebound headaches or kidney damage, use cautiously, no more than an average of two tablets a day, fourteen tablets per week, or thirty tablets a month. If more is needed, see your doctor about taking preventive medication.

SIDE EFFECTS: The caffeine may trigger anxiety and the aspirin may trigger nausea. Less common side effects include stomach pain and heartburn. Long-term or high doses can cause liver or kidney problems and stomach bleeding.

2. NAPROXEN (ALEVE)

Naproxen, which has been a prescription medication for many years, recently became available as an over-the-counter medication. It is a very effective and nonsedating medication. Coffee or a caffeine tablet may enhance its effectiveness. The prescription versions (Anaprox, Naprosyn) contain more milligrams of naproxen and are therefore stronger.

TYPICAL DOSE: One tablet (220 mg) with food or Tums or Rolaids. Total daily dose is three tablets, with eight to twelve hours between doses.

SIDE EFFECTS: Nausea and stomach upset, especially among people older than forty. With long-term daily use, liver, kidney, and gastrointestinal problems are a concern.

3. IBUPROFEN (ADVIL, HALTRAN, MEDIPREN, MIDOL 200, MOTRIN, NUPRIN, RUFEN, TRENDAR)

An inexpensive nonsteroidal anti-inflammatory (NSAID), ibuprofen is often helpful for tension and migraine headaches and reasonably well tolerated. Adding caffeine by drinking a cup of coffee or taking a caffeine pill can make the medication even more effective.

TYPICAL DOSE: From 200 (typical pill) to 800 mg every three to four hours as needed. Total dose should not exceed 2,400 mg per day, and if ibuprofen is used daily, blood tests should be taken to monitor potential liver or kidney irritation. Take with food or antacid.

SIDE EFFECTS: Commonly causes gastrointestinal upset. If you need more than an average of two pills per day, your doctor will probably recommend preventive medication.

4. ASPIRIN-FREE EXCEDRIN
Because it contains caffeine and acetaminophen only (no aspirin), it is not considered an NSAID. Without the aspirin, though, it tends to be less effective than Excedrin Extra-Strength. The lack of aspirin, however, makes it a good choice for people who tend toward ulcers, stomach upset, or excessive nausea.

TYPICAL DOSE: One or two pills every three or four hours.

SIDE EFFECTS: Seldom produces problems other than anxiety or insomnia from the caffeine.

5. ASPIRIN
Aspirin is extremely helpful in many cases and more effective than acetaminophen, but it also carries a greater risk of side effects. Avoid it during pregnancy or with gastritis or ulcer disease. It is available in many forms, including buffered, or coated, tablets.

TYPICAL DOSE: 325 to 650 mg every four hours as needed. Take with an antacid to minimize gastrointestinal irritation.

SIDE EFFECTS: Can irritate and cause bleeding of the gastrointestinal tract, thins blood and therefore prolongs bleeding time if you cut yourself, increases likelihood of bruising if you fall or bang yourself, and can cause reversible liver damage. Kidney irritation can occur with prolonged use of high doses.

6. ANACIN

Because it has less caffeine (32 mg) than Excedrin Extra-Strength, it is less effective but less likely to cause side effects or rebound headaches. It does contain plenty of aspirin: 400 mg in regular Anacin and 500 mg in Anacin Maximum-Strength.

TYPICAL DOSE: One or two tablets every three to four hours as needed. Take with food or an antacid.

SIDE EFFECTS: Because Anacin does not contain acetaminophen, it carries less risk of damage to kidneys or liver; its high level of aspirin, however, increases the risk of gastrointestinal irritation.

7. ACETAMINOPHEN

Acetaminophen is much less effective but better tolerated than aspirin or aspirin-containing products. It can be useful, however, for milder headaches, with minimal side effects, and may be used during pregnancy, with children, and with gastritis or ulcer disease.

Available in suppositories, tablets (regular and chewable), wafers, capsules, an elixir, a liquid, and as effervescent granules with sodium bicarbonate (Bromo Seltzer).

TYPICAL DOSE: One or two extra-strength tablets, 500 mg or 650 mg each, every three or four hours, limited to six pills per day. Do not exceed 4 g (4,000 mg) on any given day. If more than 1,500 mg is taken daily, rebound headaches may occur and preventive medication should be considered.

SIDE EFFECTS: If used excessively, (5 to 8 g per day, over weeks), acetaminophen may damage the kidneys, liver, and heart.

COLD AND HEAT

Reusable ice packs or wrapped ice is probably the most consistently effective nondrug therapy for headache. Ice packs help the pain by reducing swollen blood vessels. Be sure that the ice doesn't touch the skin directly but is protected with a layer of paper towel or a similar covering.

Besides applying it to the painful area, try placing it on the back of the neck, the top of the head, the forehead, temples, and so on. The earlier you use an ice pack to treat your headache, the better.

Heat (a very warm heating pad or a hot, wet washcloth) may be particularly useful during a headache to foster relaxation, increase blood flow, and relax your muscles.

Experiment to find out what feels good.

A COOL, DARK ROOM

Very often, simply taking a nap can give the brain an opportunity to get back to normal. Resting in the dark also helps because you may be particularly sensitive to light during a headache.

KEEPING A CALENDAR

So far, we've talked about ways to cope with a headache on the day it occurs. However, there are several strategies you can use to improve your headache situation in the long run. One of the most effective long-term strategies is to keep a headache worksheet for at least two months if you get frequent headaches. If you end up going to see a doctor, this will be an extremely valuable tool for assessment.

HEADACHE CALENDAR

Date	Trigger	Severity 1–10	Medication	How Well Did It Work?

If you are menstruating, mark the dates of your menstrual cycles on the calendar.

When filling in the "Trigger" column, consider the following list of triggers; they are listed in order of their importance and frequency among headache sufferers:

1. Stress
2. Weather changes

3. Hormonal changes: menstrual or premenstrual, birth control pills, pregnancy, menopause
4. Missed meal
5. Exposure to bright lights (particularly fluorescent or sun)
6. Lack of sleep
7. Foods eaten within twenty-four hours (check the list in Chapter 6)
8. Exposure to cigarette smoke
9. Exposure to perfumes or other odors
10. Letdown after stress
11. Too much sleep
12. Exercise or exertion
13. Seasonal change
14. Medications: oral contraceptives, high blood pressure medication with reserpine or hydralazine
15. Eyestrain
16. Travel by air, rail, car, bus

In the "Severity" column, enter a ranking from 1 to 10 using the following key:

1	2	3	4	5	6	7	8	9	10
mild		moderate			severe			excruciating	

PSYCHOTHERAPY AND STRESS MANAGEMENT

Although headaches are not psychological illnesses, there is little doubt that stress and anxiety can trigger the headache mechanisms that otherwise may have lain dormant and can turn a mild headache into a more severe one. Psychotherapy and stress management can teach coping skills to reduce stress. Hundreds of studies in the past decade have consistently acknowledged the power of an effective coping personality and an optimistic outlook on health. Learning how to cope and bounce back from a setback rather than imagining that it is a catastrophe really can reduce the negative effects of stress on your body and may even help you live a healthier and longer life.

ENHANCING COPING SKILLS

When you change your mind, you change your life. By changing negative attitudes and automatic, self-defeating thoughts, you can diminish stress and anxiety. You can learn to monitor negative or unproductive thoughts or behaviors and learn how to respond differently. For example, you may exaggerate a situation or imagine potential catastrophes. Thinking these thoughts makes you feel anxious, depressed, or out of control. Imagining the worst makes it difficult to concentrate on productive ways of dealing with the problem.

Learning to focus on the brighter side rather than the worst-case scenario can help you view the circumstances in perspective and prevent stress from building up.

You may want to read one of the excellent self-help books on cognitive therapy (such as *Feeling Good: The New Mood Therapy* by David D. Burns, M.D., and *Learned Optimism: How to Change Your Mind and Your Life* by Martin E. Seligman, Ph.D.) or consider working in short-term therapy with a cognitive, behavioral, or task-centered psychotherapist. These approaches, which challenge the way you think about things, can help you diminish your daily level of stress and therefore reduce the likelihood of triggering the headache response.

EXERCISE IN COPING SKILLS

INSTEAD OF THINKING THE WORST:
"I think one of my awful and debilitating headaches is starting. That means I won't get that report in on time, which will affect my performance evaluation and could even jeopardize my job! If I lose my job, I'll never be able to pay the rent."

TRY A POSITIVE THOUGHT:
"My head is starting to hurt, but I know I can deal with it. I will practice my deep breathing and take a pain reliever. I just need to relax and I'm sure it will get better."

INSTEAD OF THINKING THE WORST:
"I'm all alone in this. Everyone thinks I'm a malingerer. No one is going to believe how awful I feel."

TRY A POSITIVE THOUGHT:
"Just because my daughter got angry that I couldn't go to her soccer game again, I can't jump to the conclusion that everyone's giving up on me."

INSTEAD OF THINKING THE WORST:
"This pain is killing me. I can't take it."

TRY A POSITIVE THOUGHT:
"This is a bad headache, but I must not panic. Relaxing will make it better. Remember to breathe deeply, in and out. Relax. The more I relax, the faster the pain will subside."

By consciously avoiding the worst-case scenario and looking at the more realistic side, you can shift your point of view from feeling helpless and hopeless to feeling more in control and more resourceful. An important coping skill to learn is replacing automatic, self-defeating assumptions and interpretations with a more positive point of view.

PHYSICAL THERAPY AND CHIROPRACTIC THERAPY

Although not useful for many people, physical therapy and chiropractic manipulation can be very helpful for relieving neck tightness and pain. Both of these treatments are discussed in more detail in Chapter 13.

If you get frequent headaches that are impairing your life and ability to cope, you must consult a physician. But the techniques used by physical therapists and chiropractors can be very helpful in conjunction with other therapies.

3

. . . .

BEING A GOOD
HEALTH CONSUMER

ALTHOUGH the self-help techniques in the previous chapter are useful, they may not be powerful enough to control many of your headaches. If you get chronic or severe headaches, it is wise to discuss with a doctor how to manage your headaches and to get prescriptions for medications to treat and prevent the more severe ones.

How effectively a doctor can help you control your headaches, however, will depend a great deal on your relationship with the physician. If communication is poor, even an effective strategy will be doomed to fail. In headache treatment, finding the right combination of medications and figuring out the correct dosages takes time and mutual cooperation. Choosing the right doctor is essential. This chapter will help you:

- Prepare for a doctor's visit.
- Determine what to look for in a doctor.
- Learn to be a good healthcare consumer.
- Learn how to best communicate your headache and associated problems.
- Learn how to help the doctor most effectively help you.

BRING YOUR HEADACHE CALENDAR
TO YOUR APPOINTMENT

As we discussed in Chapter 2, having a calendar that charts a series of previous headaches will be extremely useful to the doctor in analyzing what triggers your headaches and determining the type of headaches you get. If you haven't already done so, start a headache calendar as soon as you decide to see a doctor.

CHOOSING A DOCTOR

Ironically, many of us have learned to be good consumers of appliances or automobiles, investing much time, energy, and research comparing brands, energy uses, rebates, and so on, yet relatively few of us have learned to be good healthcare consumers.

For years, consumers took a passive role, subordinate and childlike, in their relationships with their doctor. The patient blindly accepted doctor's orders without question. Yet in this age of healthcare reform, the doctor-patient relationship is becoming more balanced. Consumers need to take more responsibility to inform themselves about their condition and to track their own case and medical history. Also, as a medical consumer, you now have more rights than ever — the right to understand treatment and alternatives fully, to assess the potential benefits and risks of each alternative, and to get a second opinion.

Many physicians will treat headaches, yet not all are up-to-date about the latest techniques in headache management. To assess a doctor's knowledge about treating headaches, you might:

• Ask a nurse in the practice what percent of the doctor's clientele are headache patients.

- Ask several local physicians to recommend the best headache specialist in the area.
- Ask the doctor how effective the treatment should be in relieving the pain.
- Ask about the doctor's strategy in treating your type of headache.
- Ask about the doctor's availability after you leave the office if you have problems with a medication.

Here are some warning signs that should alert you to the need to see another practitioner. The doctor:

- Treats your headaches purely as a psychological problem.
- Minimizes the importance of your pain or expresses any doubts about your pain.
- Discourages you from bringing or presenting a prepared list of questions.
- Has inappropriately low expectations for satisfactory relief.
- Does not fully discuss with you possible risks and side effects of new medication.
- Does not create an open environment in which you feel free to express your needs, anger, and fears and to ask questions.
- Prescribes pain medication, such as Demerol or codeine, without trying a medication that aims to treat the root of the headache mechanism, such as serotonin imbalances and blood vessel changes.
- Does not encourage you to call if you experience unpleasant side effects or ineffective relief, or to schedule a follow-up visit in several weeks.

Although going to your family doctor for headache treatment may be adequate and appropriate for you, going directly to a neurologist who specializes in headaches, particularly if you think you need a comprehensive approach to your headache treatment, may save you a lot of money, time, and irritation in the long run.

If you fear that your doctor is less than fully knowledgeable about headaches, consider asking for a referral to a neurologist or a headache expert. You might say that you believe the doctor to be an outstanding internist, but every internist can't be expected to know the latest treatments for every condition. You might add that you'd like to take advantage of the recent strides in headache management, an emerging subspecialty, and state-of-the-art treatments that you understand are now available.

To ask for a second opinion, you might say, "I feel uncomfortable asking you this, but since this illness is so important to me, I need to obtain whatever information I can. I don't doubt your opinion. It's just that I need reassurance that this is the way to go. Do you have a colleague you might recommend for a consultation?"

Remember, you are the customer and need to be assertive about your own medical treatment. Free referrals can also be obtained through the headache associations listed in Appendix A.

HOW DOCTORS DO HEADACHE WORKUPS

When consulting with a doctor for headaches, be prepared to give a full medical history in as organized a way as possible. Chances are, the doctor will give you a form to fill out similar to the "Headache Intake Assessment Form" at the end of this chapter. Note that it includes the pain scale we've discussed and potential headache triggers. Use your headache calendar to fill out such a form, or attach it to the form. Before you consult with the doctor, think about how you can best describe your pain.

- Is it one-sided or two? Where about the head does it hurt (location of pain)?
- What's the typical pattern (frequency and duration of pain)? What's your headache history?
- What are your suspected triggers?

- What medications do you take for headache? How frequently? What helps? What doesn't?
- What other medications do you take?
- What's your family's history insofar as headaches are concerned? This question can be problematic, as many older people forget that they had headaches decades ago.
- How do headaches affect your daily life? work? family? social life?
- What are your patterns concerning recreation? stress reduction? How do you experience stress (in your jaw, back, head, etc.)?
- What are your past illnesses, allergies, experiences with different kinds of medications?

DESCRIBING PAIN

Be as specific as possible in describing the nature of the pain. One or more of the following may apply.

- piercing
- aching
- throbbing
- crushing
- boring
- burning
- pressing
- dull
- squeezing

Rate your pain severity as shown in Chapter 2, from 1 (very mild pain) to 10 (excruciating).

The doctor will listen to your heart, take your blood pressure, and test your nervous system through your reflexes, eye movements, and coordination. If you have a long history of migraine, tension, or cluster headache attacks that usually follow the same pattern, the doctor will be able to clearly ascertain your problem and may not suggest a head scan. Such a test may be recommended for the legal protection of the doctor. A physician could be vulnerable, for example, if a chronic headache patient ever developed a brain tumor (which would be totally unrelated to these headaches) and the court challenged the decision not to obtain a test.

Nevertheless, in assessing your headaches, the doctor will need to eliminate the possibility of serious, though rare, physical problems as the root cause of the headaches, such as sinus disease, meningitis, glaucoma, brain tumor, bleeding in the brain, fluid on the brain, stroke, high blood pressure in the brain, and so on. The doctor may ask you seemingly strange cognitive questions, such as "Can you list the months of the year backward?" or other questions to test your memory, judgment, and ability to reason. These are not psychological evaluations; rather, they are used to evaluate whether any particular area of your brain is especially affected.

Although a full medical history and physical exam can eliminate many suspicions of more serious physical problems, the doctor may also prescribe one or more of the exams in the following list.

USEFUL TESTS FOR DIAGNOSING HEAD PAIN

- **MAGNETIC RESONANCE IMAGING SCAN (MRI)**
  A noninvasive procedure, the MRI allows the doctor to detect any serious causes of the migraines in the brain. While the MRI feels very claustrophobic and is expensive, it involves no radiation and is extremely sensitive in picking up any problems in the head.
- **COMPUTERIZED AXIAL TOMOGRAPHY (CAT SCAN)**
  Also called a brain scan. This procedure can provide information on the sinuses and potential tumors or strokes. An injection of contrast dye into the arm may be necessary.

- **SINUS X-RAY**
Although an MRI or CAT scan provides more detailed information, a sinus x-ray is much less expensive.
- **SPINAL TAP**
Also called a lumbar puncture. This test is occasionally performed to assess certain nervous system conditions by evaluating the spinal fluid. It can cause a headache a few hours later. It is not necessary for most headache patients.
- **EYE PRESSURE TEST**
Also called intraocular pressure testing. An ophthalmologist does this procedure to rule out glaucoma.
- **BLOOD TESTS**
These tests can check for a variety of medical conditions, some of which may contribute to headaches, such as an abnormal thyroid.
- **ELECTROENCEPHALOGRAM (EEG)**
This procedure records the electrical patterns in the brain which can provide valuable clues to the brain's functioning. This test is painless and safe and can be particularly helpful in assessing post-traumatic (concussion) headaches.

THE RESPONSIBLE PATIENT VERSUS THE "GOOD" PATIENT

You have a choice: you can be passive and just accept a doctor's recommendations even if they prove ineffective; ignore the doctor's advice and continue to suffer in silence; or discuss openly with the doctor your concerns, even though such a discussion may be uncomfortable, and ask for a change in treatment. Some people try to be "good" for fear that the doctor will otherwise view them as "difficult." They try not to complain, ask too many questions, or admit that a medication didn't work. Yet many treatment failures are beyond anyone's control, and most doctors expect them in some patients.

Being a good patient doesn't mean being an easy patient but a fully responsible adult working with the doctor as a partner and not undermining his recommendations and working against him. As a patient, you must work to understand the problems and complexities of your case, be knowledgeable about your condition and about the medication you are going to try, and understand the strategy that your doctor is using for your headache pattern.

Your doctor can do his job best when you either follow his recommendations or explain why you didn't. Yet only half of patients actually comply with their doctors' recommendations. Worse yet, some patients don't even tell their doctors they didn't comply. Little is gained if you go to your next appointment without having followed the strategy discussed at the previous meeting; all that time between appointments is lost. Speak up or follow up by phone if you do not agree, do not understand, or have trouble following a recommendation. If you can't follow the doctor's recommendations, for whatever reason, call the office to make an alternate plan. Also, if you inconsistently or incorrectly take your medication, or take other headache-related medications at the same time without the doctor's knowledge, you can hamper treatment. The doctor can't know how to proceed properly if you didn't use the first-choice treatment rationally and correctly. Only by communicating well with the doctor can he better explain the treatment, or modify it, depending on your reaction.

You need to tell the doctor about all medications and drugs that you are taking, including over-the-counter and illegal ones.

Keep track in list form of what you've tried and what happened and keep a list of other medications you take (and the dosages) for other conditions. Bring this information to each appointment. Be sure to keep the doctor informed about other medical problems you may have.

ON BEING A GOOD HEALTH CONSUMER

Although the doctor is responsible for making proper assessments and recommendations, it is more important than ever that consumers take an active role in their own healthcare. To help prevent mistakes, track your own medical care. The doctor may, for example, prescribe a medication that could have an ill effect on an ulcer condition. Perhaps you had a problem with an ulcer some ten years ago; that information may not be on the front page of the medical chart. It's important for you to find out all you can about any new medication your doctor prescribes for you. Take responsibility by reviewing the drug information in this book or in reference books, such as the *Physicians' Desk Reference*. Standard reference books on medications, available in most public libraries, list contraindications or conditions to watch out for with each medication. Be responsible for bringing a concern from your medical history to the doctor's attention if it seems appropriate.

Also, the doctor may change the medication or dose for you over the telephone and neglect to make a notation of the change on your chart. Such mistakes happen. Doctors may also get sick or go on vacation, leaving a substitute who is unfamiliar with your case. If you can clearly convey the vital information the doctor needs, it will prove extremely helpful.

ACCEPTING ONLY SATISFACTORY RELIEF

It is your responsibility to follow up with your physician if you experience ill effects from medications and need to deviate from what the doctor prescribed. Don't give up if you come to a few dead ends. These are to be expected. It's reasonable to expect a medication to improve your headache situation from 50 to 90 percent.

HEADACHE INTAKE ASSESSMENT FORM

Name:_____

Age:_____ Sex: M F

Marital Status:_____

Name of Spouse:_____

Name(s) and age(s) of children:

_____

_____

_____

Education:_____

_____

Occupation:_____

Spouse's occupation:_____

Does anyone in your family have headaches?

_____

Have they had moderate-to-severe headaches
in the past? _____

How often do you have a moderate-to-severe
headache? _____

How long do the severe headaches last?

____ Hours   ____ One day ____ Two days

____ Three to several days

On a scale of 1 to 10, with 10 being the
worst, how severe are the headaches?

1	2	3	4	5	6	7	8	9	10
	Mild			Moderate			Severe		

How old were you when you started having
headaches? _____

Do you have some type of headache every day?

_____

How much do these daily headaches bother
you?

____ Mildly   ____ Moderately   ____ Severely

Where does the pain hurt on the daily
headaches? _____

Where does the pain hurt on the severe
headaches? _____

What kind of pain is it?
Sharp ____ Pounding ____ Aching____
Other: _____
Does your eye tear on the painful side of
your head? _____
Have the headaches been much worse in the
last few months? _____
Have the headaches been much worse in the
last year? _____
Do you frequently have nausea with these
headaches? _____ Does it bother you? ____
Do you have any visual problems, such as
flashing lights or sprinkles of light, or do
you lose your vision to one side with a
headache?_____

For women only:
Are the headaches much worse before or during the menstrual period?_____
Are you on any birth control pill or hormone? _____

Does stress play a role in the headaches?
_____

Circle any of the following factors that
play a role in your headaches or in producing an occasional headache:

Stress	Exercise
Weather changes	Missing a meal
Foods	Cigarette odor
Bright sunlight	Perfume odor
Relief from stress	Different seasons
Undersleeping	Summer
Oversleeping	Fall
Hormonal changes,	Winter
such as menstrual cycle	Spring
Exertion	Sexual activity

Do you have very cold feet and hands in the winter? _____

Have you had a CAT scan for the headaches?__
  If so, when?_____

Have you had an MRI for the headaches?_____
  If so, when?_____

Have you had blood tests in the past year?__
  Were they normal?_____

Have you had any biofeedback or relaxation training for headaches?_____
  If so, has it helped?_____

Which doctors/headache doctors, if any, have you seen for headaches?

_____

_____

_____

_____

_____

_____

_____

List medications
you have taken
for headaches.   Did it help?

_____   _____

_____   _____

_____   _____

_____   _____

_____   _____

_____   _____

_____   _____

_____   _____

_____   _____

4

················

RECOGNIZING MIGRAINES

THE TECHNIQUES we've described thus far are most appropriate for preventing mild headaches or for keeping mild headaches from turning into severe ones. But for a chronic migraine sufferer, these techniques may fall short. A better understanding of migraines and migraine treatment will be essential for you to learn how to improve your quality of life.

Migraines can be devastating, with their sweeps of pain that can wipe out your ability to function and to think. Some 12 percent of us — about 18 percent of American women and 7 percent of men — are stricken at one time or another. Responsible for up to $7 billion in absenteeism and billions more in diminished productivity and healthcare costs, migraines disrupt the lives of millions of Americans. Yet, to a great extent, these headaches remain underdiagnosed and undertreated.

WHO GETS MIGRAINES?

Most people who get migraines are probably born with a predisposition to them which has been passed down from one generation to the next. At least four out of five migraine sufferers can identify a family connection, more than the sufferers of any other type of headache. Whether a person with an inherited predisposition actually gets frequent migraines depends on whether certain triggers (foods, bright lights, and so on, as explained in Chapter 6) aggravate his system enough to reach a threshold that sets off the migraine mechanisms.

Women are the most likely victims: they get migraines three times more often than men, probably because of all the hormonal changes they undergo.

Although migraines can strike at any age, most who are afflicted have well-defined migraines by their late teens and twenties and then get daily or almost daily tension headaches with occasional migraines later in middle age. These are called "transformed migraines" and add weight to the theory that migraines and tension headaches are part of the same headache spectrum. Some researchers believe that transformed migraines may actually be rebound headaches that develop from daily or almost daily use of over-the-counter medications, which turn sporadic headaches into frequent ones.

Occasionally, migraines and other kinds of headaches do begin in one's fifties and sixties. If this is your experience, be sure to consult a physician because headaches can be a symptom of certain medical conditions that become more common with advancing age, such as certain brain disorders, arthritis, heart or kidney disease, high blood pressure, anemia, spine disorder, and respiratory illnesses. Although the chances are that the headaches do not stem from one of these problems, they should be excluded as possible causes.

One popular myth is that well-educated and wealthy people get more migraines. The truth is, these people just go to doctors more often. Lower-income women, in fact, have the highest risk of migraines, perhaps because they endure more day-to-day stress trying to make ends meet. Stress, we'll see time and again, is a powerful trigger in setting off migraines and other types of headaches.

Do people who get migraines have a certain stress-driven migraine personality? Some people think that a certain type of person — a perfectionist who is excessively critical of himself and others, and who gets angry but holds it in — is more prone to migraines. Yet most headache experts disagree. As we've said, migraines are inherited biochemical conditions or predispositions, much like asthma and heart disease, and not the result of a high-strung personality. The "gene" for migraines has been identified in several families.

WHAT ARE MIGRAINES?

Whether caused by a chromosomal defect or biochemical imbalances, migraines and their diagnoses are not clear-cut. Typically, you will get a diagnosis of migraines if you suffer from recurring moderate to severe headaches that are triggered by stress, certain foods, weather changes, smoke, hunger, fatigue, or other factors. More specifically, if you experience at least four of these features, the chances are that your headaches are migraines.

COMMON FEATURES OF MIGRAINES

- Recurrent: usually one to five times a month, but sometimes less. Last four to seventy-two hours, occasionally longer
- Triggered by a migraine-precipitating factor: stress, certain foods, weather changes, smoke, hunger, fatigue, and so on
- Sensitivity to light, regardless of head pain. Many sufferers wear sunglasses outside during all daylight hours.
- Blurred vision
- Nausea or vomiting, which sometimes eases the head pain
- Sensitivity to noise
- Tenderness about the scalp, which may linger for hours or days after the headache pain is gone
- Early-morning onset (but may be anytime)

- Throbbing, pounding, aching, or pulsating pain, usually on one side of the face or skull and often behind an eye (though sometimes the pain moves)
- Cold hands and feet (not just when a migraine occurs) and occasionally a cold nose
- Prone to motion sickness (not just when a migraine occurs)
- Dizziness or lightheadedness
- Lethargy
- Fluid retention, with weight gain. Some people start retaining fluids before an attack and gain up to six pounds, but the weight gain is temporary.
- Vertigo, occasional but potentially disabling during an attack
- Anxiety
- A sensation of burning, prickling, tingling, numbness (paresthesia), often occurring in one hand or forearm, but may be felt in the face, around the jaw, or in both arms and legs
- Diarrhea, usually mild
- Visual disturbances or hallucinations (auras)
- Stuffy or runny nose

LESS COMMON FEATURES OF MIGRAINES

- Mild loss of ability to read, write, or even speak (aphasia)
- Confusion
- Fever, or moderate increase in body temperature
- Seizures (rare)
- Loss of muscular coordination (rare)
- Temporary paralysis (rare)

Differentiating a mild migraine from a moderate or severe tension headache can be very difficult. Yet, if the headache is recurring with repeated attacks of throbbing or severe aching, the headache is usually defined as a migraine, whether there is nausea, visual disturbances, or sensitivity to light and noise.

People with a migraine often become pale and, less often,

flush. During an attack, they may also feel too hot or too cold. Sometimes, migraine sufferers experience pupil dilation or contraction, or a teary eye on the same side of the head as the pain. These are symptoms of a cluster headache, yet people with migraines often experience such aspects of cluster headaches, including the sharp pain about one eye or temple.

AURAS

When your migraine begins, you may see brightly colored lines or dots, known as an aura. Regardless of whether you have auras or not, the recommended treatment generally is the same. About 40 percent of sufferers, more commonly men, experience visual problems before or during the attack. Many people experience these auras only once or twice in a lifetime. Usually, they last fifteen to twenty minutes and may be as troublesome as the pain of the migraine. Sometimes these symptoms occur without pain, more commonly in adults over fifty. If you experience these symptoms, be sure to check with a doctor to rule out other disorders, particularly a condition called transient ischemic attack.

VISUAL DISTURBANCES
THAT MAY OCCUR WITH MIGRAINES

- Flashes of light
- Spots, stars, lines that are often wavy, color splashes, and waves resembling heat waves
- Shimmering, sparkling, or flickering images
- Mild loss in vision, with unformed hallucinations
- Dark spot in one's vision, often crescent-shaped, usually with zigzags. There is often a shimmering, sparkling, or flickering light at the edges of the dark spot.
- Graying or whiteout

PHASES OF A MIGRAINE

Migraines often occur in several stages.

WARNING

From hours to even a day before the pain begins, you may sense subtle neurological changes that are manifested by fatigue, irritability, depression, or moodiness. You may crave certain foods, yawn repeatedly, retain fluids, become more sensitive to light or sound, and be less attentive. Called the prodome, this phase occurs in about half to 80 percent of migraine sufferers. If you experience it, you can learn to recognize the early symptoms, predict an attack, and prepare.

AURA

Not everyone who gets migraines experiences this phase. Typically lasting less than an hour, the aura includes visual disturbances, and sometimes neurological ones: you may experience tingling or numbness on one side of the face or down one arm, difficulty speaking or remaining perfectly coordinated, or one of the less common features listed earlier in this chapter.

If you experience auras, your migraines are considered classic migraines; those without auras are called common migraines.

PAINFUL HEADACHE

Lasting four to seventy-two hours, this phase is characterized by moderate to severe pain, often accompanied by sharp "ice-pick jabs." Most people describe their pain as throbbing, pounding, or pulsating, although some people feel a severe ache. Other symptoms during this phase include lack of appetite, nausea, vomiting, sensitivity to light and sound, and muscle tenderness in the head and neck.

RESOLUTION

In this phase, which may or may not occur, the pain is gone but you feel completely washed out, depleted of energy or depressed, and some people may even vomit. Others, however, feel completely relieved and calm, even euphoric. Sometimes, sensations similar to the warning phase may return (changes in food habits, moodiness, and so on). In addition, your scalp may remain sensitive.

CAUSES OF MIGRAINES

Scientists still aren't sure what causes migraines. For many years, researchers believed that blood vessel spasms in the face, neck, and head caused these headaches. The theory was that the initial spasm, or tightening, reduced blood flow, which caused general discomfort and the auras; then the blood vessels became inflamed, which caused pain.

The current theory suggests that when a person's migraine triggers build up and exceed his threshold, normal neurological functioning is disrupted. If he experiences an aura, it is thought to be the result of a "spreading depression" over the brain. This is an electromagnetic or metabolic change, which has been observed in animals. It occurs like a wave and affects neurons in the brain. Changes in the blood vessels are probably the result, not the cause, of these changes in the brain.

Whether the aura occurs, scientists believe that something (perhaps dropping levels of magnesium) causes the trigeminal nerve, a large nerve that branches into the face and jaw and sends signals from the brain throughout the skull, to release small proteins called peptides. The peptides cause the surrounding blood vessels to swell, which in turn irritates surrounding nerve fibers, causing them to pulse and fire inappropriately and send pain signals deep into the brain.

More and more scientists are becoming convinced that serotonin, an essential chemical involved in communication among nerve cells, plays a key role in triggering migraines. The effectiveness of sumatriptan, one of the newest and most promising drugs, supports this theory. The medication works by binding to serotonin receptors, preventing nerve fibers from releasing their peptides, thereby quieting down the activity of the nerves and stifling their firings.

GENERAL MIGRAINE STRATEGY

Regardless of the biochemical causes of migraines, when you consult a doctor, his agenda typically will be:

- To determine whether you are getting rebound headaches from overdependence on caffeine or pain relievers and to help you get off them.
- To help you identify possible triggers, including specific foods.
- To be sure you understand the role of relaxation techniques, exercise, the use and overuse of caffeine and over-the-counter medications, and potential triggers.
- To give you an effective abortive medication, one that prevents a mild headache from worsening. These drugs work best if you have consistent warning signs even a half hour before the migraine actually starts raging. Abortive medications work either by preventing blood vessel inflammation, constricting blood vessels, blocking nerve cell pain signals, or changing the brain's blood chemistry.
- In some cases, to arm you with medication that can relieve disturbing side effects of a migraine, such as nausea or vomiting, and severe pain. These medications are pain relievers (some potentially addictive and, if misused, likely to cause rebound headaches) and antinausea medications.

- To find a daily preventive medication (one that is **not** potentially addictive) if you need abortive medication too frequently.
- To use a trial-and-error approach. The more you understand this strategy, the better you can help the doctor help you.

In other words, once the doctor ensures that you are not experiencing rebound headaches or drug dependence, he will try to prescribe medication to relieve your pain and other symptoms, with the goal of minimal medication and side effects.

Don't get frustrated if you and your doctor don't get it right the first time. Although you may feel like a guinea pig or that the doctor is stabbing in the dark, he is actually using a systematic trial-and-error approach. If you understand that approach, you will be able to make the treatment work most effectively and efficiently.

5

TREATING MIGRAINES
IN PROGRESS

IF YOU START getting a migraine, try to manage it with the techniques we describe in Chapter 2. In summary, these techniques include doing a relaxation exercise, having a caffeine drink or tablet, using an over-the-counter (OTC) pain reliever, applying ice packs, and napping in a dark room. When these techniques do not work, your doctor will probably prescribe an abortive medication, that is, a medicine used to relieve a headache in progress.

FIRST-LINE MEDICATIONS FOR MIGRAINE RELIEF

When a mild nonsteroidal anti-inflammatory (NSAID) with or without caffeine doesn't work to relieve a brewing migraine, most doctors will suggest several alternative medications that might have minimal side effects. These include stronger NSAIDs than the OTC drugs and mild blood vessel constrictors. Although there are much more effective migraine medications, especially dihydroergotamine (DHE) and sumatriptan (Imitrex), both of which help to constrict blood vessels as well as influence serotonin levels, they are not usually a doctor's first choice because milder medications with fewer side effects may work. Also, the most effective medications must be taken by injection (such as sumatriptan, available in pill form but more effective as an injection), so they are considered only when more convenient and milder medications prove to be inadequate.

Unfortunately, some doctors use heavy-duty narcotic medications just to treat the pain, rather than using a first-line medication to influence the headache mechanism itself. The narcotics are powerful medications that in most cases should be used at last resort. If migraines strike frequently, well-informed doctors will use a preventive treatment (see Chapter 6) in addition to an abortive one.

Choosing a first-line abortive medication, or deciding to jump to a second-line abortive, depends on:

- Your age. Some medications, as you'll see, should be avoided by certain age groups.
- Whether nausea occurs. If so, avoid aspirin and the nonsteroidal anti-inflammatories.
- Whether you need to work and function at optimal levels. If so, you should probably avoid the sedating medications.
- Your experience with each medication. Often one medication won't work for you but a similar one will. For someone else, the opposite may be true.

Although many of the medications described in this and subsequent chapters have not received specific approval from the Food and Drug Administration (FDA) for migraine use, they are considered reasonable, appropriate, and common treatments for headaches.

As with other descriptions of medications in this book, the information that follows is a guideline and is in no way prescriptive.

Here are some details on first-line abortive medications. The over-the-counter medications are listed here in their order of consideration, but you should refer to Chapter 2 for more information about them.

Please note: For most headache medications, particularly the "as-needed abortives," the generics do not work as well as the brand names. Although generics contain the same compounds as brand names, their binders and other substances are often less effective. As a result, brand name medications may be absorbed into the bloodstream more thoroughly.

FIRST-LINE MEDICATIONS
FOR ABORTING MIGRAINES

1. NONSTEROIDAL ANTI-INFLAMMATORIES (NSAIDs)

These are often the first medications to try if you are under seventy-five years of age. If you are over sixty-five, chances are your doctor won't recommend these drugs because older people are more sensitive to their gastrointestinal side effects. In this case, the doctor may skip to one of the butalbital compounds that are easier to tolerate.

We discussed these NSAIDs (with the exception of Anaprox DS) in detail in Chapter 2. The typical doses and side effects listed there apply to migraines as well.

- **EXCEDRIN EXTRA-STRENGTH**

  This particular OTC medication is very effective but can cause anxiety, nausea, and less often, stomach pain.

- **ASPIRIN-FREE EXCEDRIN**

  Although less effective than Excedrin Extra-Strength, this OTC drug does not cause stomach irritation, making it especially useful for people with ulcers or for those who often get nauseated.

- **NAPROXEN (ANAPROX DS, ALEVE)**

  A very effective, nonsedating medication that unfortunately often causes stomach upset, especially in people over forty. That's why doctors usually recommend that you accompany naproxen with food or an antacid. This drug is particularly useful for menstrual migraines and is commonly used as a preventive medication (see Chapter 6). Naproxen is available over the counter in 200 mg tablets. Anaprox DS (double-strength) tablets contain 550 mg. Coffee or a caffeine tablet may enhance its effectiveness.

TYPICAL DOSE: One tablet (Anaprox DS) with food or a Tums or Rolaids to start. If you do not experience any serious nausea, repeat in one hour, and then in three or four hours. Three-per-day maximum.

SIDE EFFECTS: Nausea and stomach upset, especially among older people. (To relieve nausea, metoclopramide (Reglan) or promethazine (Phenergan) is often prescribed to take before the naproxen.) With long-term daily use, liver, kidney, and gastrointestinal problems are a concern.

- **IBUPROFEN (ADVIL, HALTRAN, MEDIPREN, MIDOL 200, MOTRIN, NUPRIN, RUFEN, TRENDAR)**
These are inexpensive over-the-counter NSAIDs that are occasionally helpful and reasonably well tolerated, although they cause stomach upset in some people. Adding caffeine, either with coffee or in pill form, often enhances their effectiveness.

2. MIDRIN

Midrin, a combination of a blood vessel constrictor (isometheptene mucate), a mild sedative with no addiction potential (dichloralphenazone), and acetaminophen, is extremely effective and well tolerated. It can be prescribed for children as young as five and is safe with the elderly as well.

Although Midrin may cause fatigue, taking it with caffeine (either strong coffee or 50 to 100 mg of caffeine, as found in No Doz) can counter this effect while at the same time enhancing the drug's overall effectiveness.

TYPICAL DOSE: One or two capsules when headache begins, then one capsule every hour as needed but no more than six per day or twenty per week.

The first time you try Midrin, take only one capsule because fatigue or lightheadedness may be overwhelming with two.

For children or others who have difficulty swallowing the large capsule, pull it apart and spread the contents in applesauce or yogurt. This method may also be used when only half a capsule is needed.

Generic Midrin is not as effective as brand name.

SIDE EFFECTS: Generally well tolerated, but fatigue or mild stomach upset is common. Occasional lightheadedness. Can raise blood pressure so is used with great caution among those with high blood pressure.

3. NORGESIC FORTE

This medication consists of a relatively large dose of aspirin (770 mg) and caffeine (60 mg) coupled with a nonaddicting muscle relaxant (50 mg of orphenadrine), which is also an antihistamine. It is considered one of the more potent nonaddictive analgesics for getting rid of a migraine.

TYPICAL DOSE: One-half to one pill every three hours as needed but no more than four a day. These pills are large so you may want to break them in half for easier swallowing. Be sure to take with food or an antacid.

SIDE EFFECTS: Fatigue, lightheadedness, upset stomach, are common. If nausea occurs, talk to your doctor about trying an aspirin-free medication. The high aspirin content may also cause stomach pain. The muscle relaxant in Norgesic Forte occasionally causes blurred vision.

4. BUTALBITAL COMPOUNDS

All these medications are potentially addicting because of the butalbital, a barbiturate sedative, but they are considered safe and effective when used sparingly.

• FIORINAL

This drug is the most effective of the butalbital compounds because it contains aspirin instead of acetaminophen; it also contains caffeine and butalbital. Many people experience a brief high or euphoria with the medication, however, and this effect can lead to addiction. It is important not to take it, therefore, to relieve stress and anxiety.

TYPICAL DOSE: One or two pills every three hours as needed, but should not be taken more than two days a week; no more than forty pills per month. Occasionally, use of one or two on a daily basis is justified.

SIDE EFFECTS: Fatigue, lightheadedness, nausea, and euphoria are relatively common. Anxiety or rebound headaches occur occasionally. When taken for anxiety or stress, may lead to abuse.

- **FIORINAL WITH CODEINE, FIORICET WITH CODEINE**
Though more effective than Fiorinal in relieving a migraine, the codeine causes more side effects. A major concern of using this medication is its potential for abuse.

TYPICAL DOSE: One capsule every three hours, or two every four hours, as needed.

SIDE EFFECTS: Fatigue, lightheadedness, and nausea are common. Many people can't tolerate the codeine; stomach upset or abdominal pain are fairly common.

- **FIORICET, ESGIC, AND ESGIC PLUS**
These medications are particularly useful if aspirin nauseates you because Fioricet, Esgic, and Esgic Plus contain acetaminophen instead (Esgic Plus contains additional acetaminophen). Otherwise, these drugs are similar to Fiorinal (in that they contain caffeine and butalbital). This substitution of acetaminophen for aspirin makes these medications less effective but also less troublesome, especially regarding nausea.

TYPICAL DOSE: One or two pills every three hours, as needed. Each Esgic Plus pill contains 500 mg acetaminophen; no one should consume more than 4 g (4,000 mg) daily.

SIDE EFFECTS: Fatigue and lightheadedness are most common; occasional nervousness; nausea is uncommon but may occur. To avoid addiction, these medications are usually not taken for daily headaches.

• **PHRENILIN**

Phrenilin is similar to Esgic but has no caffeine; it contains butalbital and acetaminophen. (Phrenilin Forte contains extra acetaminophen.) Although less effective than Fiorinal or Esgic, Phrenilin is useful for people who can't tolerate caffeine or aspirin or who take medication at night when they want to sleep. Many doctors recommend using Fiorinal or Esgic in the morning or afternoon and Phrenilin at night.

TYPICAL DOSE: One or two pills every three hours, as needed.

SIDE EFFECTS: Fatigue is most common because this medication has no caffeine to offset it. Occasional lightheadedness.

SECOND-LINE MEDICATIONS
FOR ABORTING MIGRAINES

If the first-line medications are not appropriate for you or have proven ineffective, a doctor may recommend one of these second-line medications.

1. SUMATRIPTAN (IMITREX)

A relatively new but expensive ($34 per injection) medication, sumatriptan is extremely effective, perhaps the most effective migraine medication with minimal side effects (nausea in some people). Tablets are available, but sumatriptan injections are far more effective. The medication comes in easy-to-use prefilled syringes with an auto-injector. The needle is small and you never actually see it. You simply press the applicator against your leg or arm and push a button. Sometimes the injection area burns, but a cold compress before the injection can help.

Although it works swiftly (sixty minutes after pills, ten to thirty minutes after injection), it lasts only about five hours and many people need another injection or a pain reliever within six to twelve hours. Using sumatriptan does carry the risk of rebound headaches (unlike DHE, dihydroergotamine, a related but older drug that is less effective but lasts longer).

Sumatriptan works differently from other headache medications. It modulates serotonin in the brain, relieving nerve inflammation in the brain's casing and perhaps constricting blood vessels in the brain.

Sumatriptan is not a good choice for children; pregnant women; women who are nursing; people with liver, kidney, or heart disease; or those over sixty years of age. While many adolescents have received sumatriptan, it has not yet been approved for this age group. People with risk factors for heart problems must have their heart checked prior to using sumatriptan.

TYPICAL DOSE: One pill (100 mg) or one injection (6 mg). If ineffective, then a pain medication (such as Fiorinal) should be taken an hour or two later. If the sumatriptan relieves the pain but the pain recurs, then an additional pill or injection may be taken, up to three tablets or two injections in a twenty-four-hour period.

SIDE EFFECTS: Nausea (although sumatriptan can also relieve the nausea of a migraine), fatigue, lightheadedness, and dizziness. People often describe feeling a rush in their head, or a brief period of increased headache. Tingling, heat flashes, and feelings of pressure or heaviness in any part of the body may also occur. Chest heaviness is common, but is believed to be unrelated to the heart.

2. DHE (DIHYDROERGOTAMINE)

In addition to constricting arterial blood vessels mildly, DHE probably works by also modulating serotonin. This medication is safe, very well tolerated, and very effective if you are willing to give yourself an injection (it is not available in premeasured auto-injectors so you must draw the medication up into a syringe). It is not quite as effective as sumatriptan but lasts longer and carries no risk of rebound headaches. It is expensive, however, and is available only as an injection or nasal spray (less effective than the injection).

DHE is not a good choice for people who are pregnant; have angina, poorly controlled high blood pressure, or poor circulation in their hands or feet; or are over age sixty.

TYPICAL DOSE: As an injection, 1 mg (one vial) is typical, but 0.5 to 1.5 mg is not uncommon. As a nasal spray, one spray in each nostril to start, which may be repeated. Although DHE does not cause rebound headaches, 5 mg in a week should be the limit, five injections or twelve nasal sprays. DHE may be used for two days in a row.

SIDE EFFECTS: Although there are many possible side effects, they are unlikely to last more than a day, and serious side effects are very rare. Most side effects last less than an hour.

Nausea is very common, so it's often a good idea to take antinausea medication (such as Reglan, Compazine, Tigan, or Phenergan) about ten minutes before you take DHE. If you get stomach upset or heartburn but no nausea, try an antacid like Rolaids or Tums.

Flushed feeling or heat in the head, leg cramps or aching in the legs, are common sensations. The nasal spray can cause nasal congestion.

Muscle tension, mild headache, tightness in the chest or throat, may occur briefly. Numbness or burning at the injection site may be prevented by icing the area before the injection. Diarrhea lasting about a day may occur, especially with intravenous administration.

3. ERGOTAMINES
These medications are often effective because they effectively constrict blood vessels that have become abnormally dilated.

But they often cause many side effects, including nausea and anxiety. If these medications are overused, the resulting rebound headaches can be severe. People over forty should use ergotamine with caution because this drug increases the risk of heart attack.

• **CAFERGOT PILLS**

These are among the most commonly used ergotamines because they may be taken orally and are thus more convenient than their suppository counterparts; they are, however, the least effective of this group. They must not be used more than one day in four to avoid the risk of rebound headaches.

TYPICAL DOSE: One or two pills when pain begins, repeating every half hour or hour; no more than five a day or ten a week. When used two days in a row, rebound headache may result.

SIDE EFFECTS: Nausea with occasional vomiting is common. Nervousness, difficulty sleeping, and dizziness may occur. Less common are numbness, tingling, or muscle pain in the fingers or toes.

• **CAFERGOT SUPPOSITORIES**

Though less convenient than pills, these suppositories, which contain caffeine and ergotamine, are much more effective. They're usually not a good choice, however, if you tend to get diarrhea with your migraine.

TYPICAL DOSE: Starting with one-third to half a suppository, the dose may be adjusted up or down depending on the patient's response. No more than two per day, one in four days, or four per week is recommended.

SIDE EFFECTS: Same as for the Cafergot pills but with less nausea.

• **CAFERGOT PB SUPPOSITORIES**

More effective with fewer side effects than suppositories without pentobarbital but not as widely available. A generic preparation is available, and certain pharmacists can prepare these suppositories themselves. Cafergot PB Suppositories contain caffeine, ergotamine, and pentobarbital, which can cause sedation but helps reduce nausea.

TYPICAL DOSE: Same as for the Cafergot Suppositories without pentobarbital.

SIDE EFFECTS: Same as for the Cafergot Suppositories without pentobarbital but significantly milder. Sedation, however, is more common with this preparation.

4. KETOROLAC (TORADOL)

Ketorolac is a moderately effective anti-inflammatory. It's a good choice when you want to reduce risk of sedation or addiction or if you can't take medication orally because you tend to vomit with your migraines. Like many other medications, this drug is more effective when injected than when swallowed in pill form. The injections are available in convenient, prefilled syringes, but the needle is large.

TYPICAL DOSE: When injected, 60 mg is a typical dose, which may be repeated in an hour if needed. No more than 120 mg per day, only once a week.

SIDE EFFECTS: Stomach upset or pain, occasional sedation. Possible liver or kidney problems; people with any liver or kidney impairments should not take ketorolac; older people should use it very cautiously.

5. CORTICOSTEROIDS

Cortisone (either pill or injection) is one of the most effective medications for severe, prolonged migraines and menstrual migraines, but it can only be taken in small doses and for brief periods of time. Long-term use of cortisone can cause serious side effects, such as weight gain, adrenal gland suppression, and predisposition to fractures and liver failure.

Dexamethasone (Decadron) and Prednisone are oral medications; Depo-Medrol or ACTH (adrenocorticotropic hormone) are administered by injection.

TYPICAL DOSE: One tablet, 20 mg Prednisone or 4 mg Decadron, taken with food, and repeated every four to six hours as needed. No more than three tablets per month. None of the corticosteroids should be taken with NSAIDs or gastrointestinal bleeding can occur.

When migraines are triggered by flying, a half or whole Decadron or Prednisone pill should be taken a half hour before flight time. For altitude migraines, take one pill a half hour to an hour before your plane arrives in a high-altitude city or before you reach a high summit. Take another pill four hours later. Dose can be repeated for two days.

For severe, prolonged migraines, Depo-Medrol injections (40 to 80 mg) or ACTH gel (40 to 80 units) may help, but limit to once per two months at most.

SIDE EFFECTS: Possibly nausea, insomnia, stomach upset, nervousness, and facial flushing. Occasional weight gain or water retention. More rarely, fatigue or agitation.

6. NARCOTICS AND SEDATIVES

When sumatriptan, DHE, ergotamine, ketorolac, or one of the corticosteroids doesn't help or causes too many side effects, a stronger narcotic, usually given with an antinausea medication, may be the answer. Doctors may be somewhat more reluctant to use these medications because of their potential for nausea as well as for abuse that can lead to addiction. Typically, these medications can calm you and induce sleep. They are useful only for one to three days and shouldn't be used every day unless every other method for controlling daily headaches has failed.

• MILD NARCOTICS

The milder narcotics, or opioids, can be taken by mouth.

– ACETAMINOPHEN WITH CODEINE (TYLENOL 3, WITH 30 MG CODEINE, AND TYLENOL 4, WITH 60 MG CODEINE) has no aspirin and therefore induces less nausea.

- **EMPIRIN WITH CODEINE** contains aspirin (which is good for migraines) and codeine, but also tends to induce nausea.
- **HYDROCODONE WITH ACETAMINOPHEN (VICODIN, HYDROCET, AND LORCET)** is well tolerated for a narcotic medication.
- **PROPOXYPHENE (DARVON OR DARVOCET)** is sometimes helpful for migraine sufferers when the first three mild narcotics aren't. As with many medications, each person responds differently.

    TYPICAL DOSE: One or two pills every three or four hours, as needed.

    SIDE EFFECTS: Nausea, sedation, addiction.

• **STRONG NARCOTICS**

Sometimes these strong medications are the only ones that will help a severe migraine. No more than three or four tablets a day or ten pills a month for any of these medications is recommended. Injections offer better pain relief than tablets and may be administered with an antinausea medication.

- **MEPERIDINE (DEMEROL)** injections are more effective than tablets.

    TYPICAL DOSE: For oral meperidine, 50 to 100 mg every three to four hours, as needed; 50 to 125 mg per injection.

    SIDE EFFECTS: Nausea and drowsiness, sometimes constipation. Can be habit-forming if used often.

- **METHADONE (DOLOPHINE)** lasts longer than Demerol and carries less potential for nausea and addiction.

    TYPICAL DOSE: 5 or 10 mg per injection, every three to four hours.

    SIDE EFFECTS: Same as with meperidine.

- **OXYCODONE (PERCOCET, PERCODAN, TYLOX)**

    TYPICAL DOSE: One tablet (5 mg oxycodone with aspirin or acetaminophen) every three to four hours. Injections are not available.

    SIDE EFFECTS: Same as with meperidine.

– MORPHINE

TYPICAL DOSE: For tablets, 15 mg every three to four hours, or 10-to-15-mg injections.

SIDE EFFECTS: Same as with meperidine.

• **SEDATIVES**

Sedatives are always useful for severe migraine because sleep is a powerful weapon against headache.

– BENZODIAZEPINES

• **DIAZEPAM (VALIUM)**

A sedative and a muscle relaxant, Valium is less effective as a generic.

TYPICAL DOSE: 5 or 10 mg every three or four hours if necessary but no more than 20 mg a day. Should not be used daily.

SIDE EFFECTS: Sedation, disorientation, and euphoria; may increase depression if used frequently.

• **CLONAZEPAM (KLONOPIN)**

A somewhat stronger sedative than Valium, Klonopin is often used to induce sleep. It should not be used daily unless other means have not been helpful.

TYPICAL DOSE: 0.5 mg to 2 mg every three or four hours, as needed. No more than 4 mg a day.

SIDE EFFECTS: Drowsiness, sedation, and fatigue. Flulike withdrawal symptoms may occur if medication is used for a long time and then suddenly stopped.

PHARMACIST PREPARATIONS

Many pharmacists can prepare these and other medications not otherwise commercially available.

• **SUPPOSITORIES**

For patients too nauseated to take a pill. Many kinds of mixes are available, such as a pain reliever with an antinausea medication.

• **LOZENGES**
Particularly good for children who won't swallow pills but also useful for combining a pain reliever with an antinausea medication.

• **NASAL SPRAY**
A more convenient form of DHE than injection. DHE nasal spray has just recently become commercially available, so if your pharmacy still does not carry it, ask a "compounding" pharmacist to prepare it.

ANTINAUSEA MEDICATION

Nausea may occur not only as a side effect of a migraine, but as a side effect of medication as well. If you are susceptible to nausea, you may want to keep some antinausea medication on hand. Most of these drugs are sedating, which many migraine sufferers find helpful. The pills are less effective than the suppositories, which are less effective than injections you can give yourself. If you experience severe nausea, keep both pills and suppositories on hand.

1. OVER-THE-COUNTER ANTACIDS, VITAMIN B$_6$, OR EMETROL
These preparations are available without a doctor's prescription and include antacids such as Tums, Rolaids, or Mylanta. They can sometimes help settle your stomach during a migraine.

Vitamin B$_6$ occasionally helps, but limit yourself to one tablet a day.

Emetrol, an over-the-counter antinausea medication, may help alleviate migraine nausea. It is a phosphorated carbohydrate solution (also called Calm-X, Naus-a-way, and Nauseatol). One or two tablets every three or four hours, as needed, are usually recommended.

2. PROMETHAZINE (PHENERGAN)

Though mild and effective, promethazine can have a strong sedative effect and will often make you fall asleep; this effect, however, may be just what you want. Safe for children, the medication may cause sudden, involuntary jerking movements (extrapyramidal side effects), but they are temporary and rare and shouldn't cause concern. Promethazine is available as a pill or a suppository, and some pharmacists will make them into oral lozenges.

TYPICAL DOSE: 25 to 50 mg by mouth or in a suppository, every three to four hours, as needed.

SIDE EFFECTS: In addition to fatigue, promethazine occasionally makes you feel dizzy or lowers your blood pressure.

3. PROCHLORPERAZINE (COMPAZINE)

Compazine is a very effective antinausea medication but produces side effects — somewhat more frequently than the other antinausea medications.

In addition to being available in long-acting pill form and suppositories, Compazine can also be taken intravenously and sometimes helps to relieve pain.

TYPICAL DOSE: 10 to 25 mg by mouth, 5 or 25 mg in suppositories, or 5 to 10 mg by injection, every three to four hours, but no more than 60 mg a day.

SIDE EFFECTS: Involuntary movements, anxiety and agitation, fatigue.

4. METOCLOPRAMIDE (REGLAN)

Because Reglan is well tolerated, with only mild side effects, it is commonly used before IV DHE, which may be given in an emergency room for quick relief of severe pain.

TYPICAL DOSE: 5 to 10 mg every four hours, as needed, but no more than 30 mg a day.

SIDE EFFECTS: Mild fatigue or anxiety and restlessness, occasional involuntary jerking.

5. TRIMETHOBENZAMIDE (TIGAN, ARRESTIN, BENZACOT, BIO-GAN, STEMETIC, TEBAMIDE, TEGAMIDE, TICON, TIGECT-20, TRIBAN, TRIBENZAGAN)

Tigan is somewhat less effective than the other antiemetics (antinausea medications) but may be prescribed for children and has few and minimal side effects.

Tigan is available in pills and suppositories, and some pharmacists will make oral lozenges.

TYPICAL DOSE: 250 mg by mouth or as a suppository or injection, every three hours, as needed.

SIDE EFFECTS: Fatigue; occasional involuntary jerking, dizziness, blurred vision, and low blood pressure.

6. CHLORPROMAZINE (THORAZINE, PROMAPAR, SONAZINE)

Although this medication is the most effective one for relieving nausea, it has more side effects than other antiemetics and is usually reserved for when they fail. The medication also helps with pain, however, and the suppositories can often prevent a trip to the emergency room by sedating you, inducing sleep, and thereby stopping the nausea.

TYPICAL DOSE: 25 to 50 mg by mouth or in a suppository, every three hours, as needed.

SIDE EFFECTS: Long-lasting sedation. May also cause dizziness and, occasionally, involuntary jerking and slurred speech.

7. ONDANSETRON (ZOFRAN)

This relatively new antinausea medication, used primarily for cancer patients receiving chemotherapy, is effective, with remarkably few side effects. It rarely causes the sedation that the other antinausea medications bring on. However, it is expensive, at $8 to $12 per tablet.

TYPICAL DOSE: One tablet (4 or 8 mg) every six to eight hours, as needed.

SIDE EFFECTS: Though rare, nervousness, diarrhea, or constipation may occur.

CASE STUDIES

Here are two sample case studies to show you how a doctor might manage occasional migraines with abortive medications. Although many cases are simple, we have chosen two complex ones to take you through the rational trial-and-error process that a headache doctor might use.

ERIC

INITIAL VISIT: Eric, a hard-driving executive, is forty-three years old and has had migraines for twelve years. His father and grandfather also had migraines. He is a perfectionist in his work and suffers from very cold hands and feet. He has a history of motion sickness as a child, and his eyes are very sensitive to light.

Eric reports that none of the over-the-counter medications have helped his migraines, which are so severe that they keep him from functioning. Because he suffers from only two a month, Eric's doctor does not place him on daily preventive medication. However, because his migraines are severe, last two days, and are accompanied by nausea and vomiting, they discuss daily preventive medication as a possibility for the future. (Patients who find such medication worthwhile usually have four to five migraines a month or chronic daily tension headaches.)

The doctor first briefs Eric on the importance of relaxation methods. Then he prescribes Compazine suppositories for the nausea and DHE nasal spray and butalbital with caffeine and acetaminophen (Esgic) for the headaches. The generic painkillers (generic Esgic, for example) do not work as well as the brand names.

WEEK 1: Eric calls to say that he is nervous and agitated, so the doctor changes his nausea medication from Compazine to promethazine (Phenergan), which is more sedating but does not cause nervousness.

WEEK 3: Eric comes in and reports that the DHE is not useful, but the butalbital compound does relieve the headache pain to a small extent. The doctor prescribes sumatriptan (Imitrex) to replace the DHE and teaches Eric how to inject himself.

WEEK 4: Eric calls to say the sumatriptan works to stop his headache for eleven hours, at which time the headache returns and he takes another injection (as he was told he could do). The doctor then prescribes a small amount of dexamethasone (Decadron), a cortisone medication, which can be very useful in shortening migraines that tend to last for two or more days.

WEEK 6: Eric reports good control of his migraines. The sumatriptan injections relieve the headache, and the dexamethasone effectively prevents it from returning. The promethazine continues to work well for nausea.

THE FUTURE: If Eric later reports that he is losing control of his headaches, other possibilities for him include ergotamines, DHE injections, Midrin, and Norgesic Forte. A daily preventive medication is also a consideration.

ROBIN

INITIAL VISIT: Robin is a thirty-nine-year-old lawyer who gets severe migraines about twice a month; they last for two days each. She gets no relief from various over-the-counter medications and relaxation-biofeedback methods. With previous physicians, she tried naproxen (Anaprox) and Norgesic Forte, neither of which were particularly helpful. The migraines are triggered occasionally by weather changes or stress, but 80 percent of the time the headaches do not have any identifiable trigger (as is the case for most people). Visits to a chiropractor, massage therapist, and acupuncturist have failed to provide any relief. Robin is very reluctant to use a daily preventive medication. She simply wishes to treat the headaches once they occur with an abortive medication.

Robin's doctor first instructs her on basic nonmedication

techniques such as lying down in a dark room and applying ice packs to her head. He prescribes Midrin and Fiorinal and tells Robin to try them separately and together.

WEEK 3: Robin reports that these medications separately give her only about 20 percent relief; when she combines them she gets slightly more relief, but the combination fatigues her. Robin's doctor prescribes sumatriptan (Imitrex) instead and teaches her how to do self-injections.

WEEK 6: Robin calls to say that the Imitrex stops the migraine within forty-five minutes but causes chest tightness and nausea that pass within twenty minutes. She says the relief lasts only eight hours. The doctor tells her to try another injection when the headache recurs. Robin does, and then calls to say that the relief from the second injection lasts three to four hours. Since the injections are costly, Robin says she can't afford more than four injections per month, allowing her two injections per migraine.

The doctor also prescribes dexamethasone (Decadron), a cortisone preparation that helps shorten severe prolonged migraines. The dose should be limited, so the prescription includes only three pills per month. The Decadron is very helpful in shortening the migraine to one day and for that one day, the Imitrex provides good relief.

SIX MONTHS LATER: Robin comes in because the Imitrex has "worn out" and is no longer effective. This phenomenon occurs with many medications, although some people can rely on the same medicine for years. Robin's doctor now prescribes dihydroergotamine (DHE) injections to use at home, which are somewhat less effective and less expensive than Imitrex but longer-lasting. She continues on the Decadron to shorten the migraines.

WEEK 2: Robin calls to say the DHE was helpful but produced a lot of nausea. The doctor prescribes ergotamine with caffeine (Cafergot) in pill form instead and tells her to continue the Decadron as well.

WEEK 4: The Cafergot pills provide relief, but Robin is still getting too nauseated. The doctor replaces the pills with Cafergot suppositories (one-half suppository to be used every four to six hours as needed) because they generally produce less nausea and are more effective than the tablets.

WEEK 7: The suppositories are somewhat effective, but the nausea is still a problem. The doctor then prescribes generic Cafergot PB suppositories (to be formulated by a compounding pharmacist), which help to reduce the nausea. In combination with the Decadron, these suppositories relieve her severe pain and limit the migraines to one day or less.

THE FUTURE: If Robin needs to try other abortive medications, hydrocodone, Fiorinal with codeine, or meperidine are possibilities; she may also try Imitrex again in the future. Because she gets only two migraines a month, she does not necessarily need preventive medication, although some patients who get two severe and prolonged migraines a month find them worthwhile. If Robin decides in the future to give preventives a try, she may start with one of the medications that we discuss in the next chapter, amitriptyline (Elavil), propranolol (Inderal), or verapamil (Isoptin, Calan, or Verelan).

6

. . . .

PREVENTING MIGRAINES

IT'S ONE THING to have mastered the techniques for bailing yourself out of a migraine if one starts, but an important long-term goal is learning how to prevent your migraines *before* they start. One way to achieve this goal is to identify which triggers most affect you. Another is to take a preventive medication if you get migraines frequently.

To use this chapter most efficiently, track your migraines with the Headache Calendar in Chapter 2. Every time a headache comes on, try to identify which factor on the list might have played a role in triggering it. Highlight a handful of potential triggers and do all you can to eliminate them from your life. See if the headaches improve. Reintroduce the potential triggers one at a time. Later in this chapter, we will discuss preventive medications to use when the nondrug strategies don't work well enough.

RECOGNIZING COMMON TRIGGERS

Many factors have been identified as possible migraine triggers, but most people are sensitive to only a few. Unfortunately, however, what triggers a headache today won't necessarily be what brings one on next week. Also, the different elements to which you are sensitive can gang up and give you a terrible headache even when they might not have affected you individually. A sudden weather change compounded by job stress, for example, may be enough to take you over the edge. Not everyone can isolate the primary headache culprits, but others, through experience, do notice specific patterns. The more observant you are in identifying your patterns, the better off you'll be. Be mindful of these potential triggers:

COMMON MIGRAINE TRIGGERS

- Stress, worry, depression, anxiety, and anger
- Some foods
- Weather and seasonal changes, such as high humidity or high heat
- Smoke, perfume, gasoline, paint, organic solvents, and other strong odors
- Hunger
- Fatigue or lack of sleep
- Hormonal factors, such as menstruation, birth control pills, pregnancy, menopause, estrogens
- Oversleeping and excessive sleep
- Exertion, exercise, or sex
- Bright lights, such as glaring artificial lights or bright sunlight
- Head trauma
- Altitude
- Motion, experienced during long car rides or amusement park rides, for example

STRESS, WORRY, DEPRESSION, ANXIETY, AND ANGER

Although emotions do not *cause* migraines, which are an inherited, physical illness, certain emotions can *trigger* migraines. Any problem — trouble at work, illness in the family, financial woes, bickering with a loved one — that causes stress may bring on a headache. That's not to say that the headache is psychological; rather, the stress causes complex biochemical changes in the body that can disrupt your equilibrium, cause your neck, shoulders, and head muscles to tighten up, thereby triggering your susceptible headache mechanism.

For some people, stress itself triggers a migraine. In others, however, the letdown period that occurs after a stressful event or period precipitates a headache. Monday-to-Friday workers, for example, often suffer from weekend headaches. Migraine-free through the workweek, they may suffer from a letdown headache as soon as the weekend begins and the stressful week is over. Weekend headaches, as we've discussed, may also be due to caffeine withdrawal.

Depression may trigger migraines, but again, it does not cause them. As you may have experienced, suffering from severe, recurring head pain can be depressing. Recent studies have suggested that if you get migraines, you may also be at greater risk for depression and anxiety, probably because all these conditions are related to the neurotransmitter serotonin. As a result, if you do get depressed or emotionally stressed, chances are your headaches will continue until these problems are resolved.

A most effective way to resolve troubling emotions is with psychotherapy, which can teach you how to deal better with problems and to use relaxation methods to help mitigate the potentially damaging effects of stress. By helping you learn how to resolve conflicts with other people, modify perfectionist behavior, and deal with anger and other repressed emotions, you may actually find that your migraines diminish in intensity and frequency.

So don't be offended if your doctor suggests psychotherapy; such a recommendation does not imply that the pain is all in your head. Rather, he is aware of the potential yet vast benefits of psychotherapy and stress management. Too few people put in the time, effort, and money necessary to try just a few sessions with a psychotherapist to learn specific coping and relaxation skills, which can be a powerful ally in their fight against headaches. (These strategies and techniques are discussed in detail in Chapter 2.)

SOME FOODS

More than 25 percent of migraine sufferers can identify foods that trigger an attack. Note that if a specific food provokes a headache in you, this reaction is probably not an allergic one, contrary to the views of many consumers, but rather a sensitivity to specific chemicals in these foods: amines (in aged cheese, pickled herring, and bananas); phenylethylamine (in chocolate); monosodium glutamate, or MSG (in Chinese food); and nitrites (in luncheon meats, bacon, and hot dogs). The chemical may trigger a migraine because of its effect on the brain or blood vessels, which is very different from an allergic reaction.

Although food-triggered headaches often start soon after eating, several hours may go by before onset. Also, you may be sensitive to the offending food only sometimes. Women, for example, may be particularly sensitive around their menstrual periods. And remember, triggers are "additive"; one food may not cause a headache, but two offending foods may.

Study the food list that follows, and if you have a hunch about certain foods to avoid, omit them from your diet for at least several weeks. If you have no idea where to start, avoid them all or choose a few. Gradually add back one food at a time, noting which ones may be headache culprits. Don't become frustrated or disappointed if you watch the foods carefully but still get headaches. Food is but one of many influencing factors and, compared to stress and biochemical imbalances, a relatively minor one.

COMMON MIGRAINE FOOD TRIGGERS

- Alcohol (less than the amount consumed to cause a hangover), most commonly red wine, as well as brandy, whiskey, champagne, white wine, beer, and other drinks. Vodka is the least likely alcohol to trigger a migraine.
- Chocolate and chocolate milk, cocoa
- Cheese, ripened, such as Cheddar, blue, brick, Colby, Roquefort, Brie, Gruyère, mozzarella, Parmesan, Boursault, and Romano; and process, though American cheese, along with cottage cheese and cream cheese, is much less likely to trigger a headache than the aged cheeses.
- Citrus fruit, including grapefruit and orange
- Pineapple
- Caffeine in coffee, soda, cocoa, and other drinks (Usually caffeine helps headaches; too much caffeine, though, can cause increased, rebound headaches. Heavy caffeine users need to reduce their intake gradually. Some migraine sufferers are extremely sensitive to small amounts of caffeine.)
- Monosodium glutamate (MSG), may also be labeled "autolyzed yeast extract," "hydrolyzed vegetable protein," or "natural flavoring." Possible sources of MSG include Chinese restaurant food; broth or stock; canned or instant soup; whey protein; soy extract; malt extract; caseinate; barley extract; textured soy protein; chicken, pork, or beef flavoring; processed meat; smoke flavor; spices and seasonings including seasoned salt; carrageenan; meat tenderizer; TV dinners; instant gravy; and some potato chips and dry-roasted nuts.
- Hot dog, pepperoni, bologna, salami, sausage, canned or aged meat, cured meat (bacon, ham), or marinated meat
- Fresh, hot homemade yeast bread (once cool it is OK)
- Buttermilk
- Yeast extract

- Acidophilus milk
- Pizza, freshly baked and still hot (less likely to trigger headache if cooled and reheated)
- Aspartame, such as NutraSweet, a popular artificial sweetener

LESS COMMON MIGRAINE FOOD TRIGGERS

- Onion
- Beans, such as lima, navy, fava, lentil, garbanzo, pinto, and Italian
- Snow peas
- Sauerkraut
- Pickles and pickled food
- Marinades
- Chili peppers
- Licorice or carob candy
- Fig, raisin, avocado, banana, passion fruit, papaya
- Fried food
- Peanut, peanut butter
- Popcorn
- Nuts or seeds, all types
- Soy sauce
- Sugar in excess
- Salt in excess
- Seafood
- Sour cream or yogurt
- Pork and chicken liver

WEATHER AND SEASONAL CHANGES

Spring tends to be the worst season for migraine sufferers, then fall. The hot humid days of summer may also be bad. You may be sensitive to weather changes, regardless of the season. Weather tends to affect the severity, not the frequency, of migraines. Although research on weather and headache produces conflicting results, more often than not weather emerges as a major trigger. However, most weather triggers for migraines can't be pinpointed to any single identifiable cause.

SMOKE, PERFUME, GASOLINE, PAINT, ORGANIC SOLVENTS

Certain people are particularly sensitive to these substances. Sensitivity to cigarette smoke may develop anytime, even in people who used to be smokers. Many people cannot stand to be exposed to even small amounts of perfumes or gasoline. Magazines that contain perfume are often a hazard for the migraine-prone (subscription magazines may be ordered without them); paint smells are also common triggers for migraines.

HUNGER

Most people who get migraines recognize that if they miss meals they are more likely to get a headache. If this is true for you, be sure to eat regularly, at least three times a day. Anticipate periods when there may not be food available (when traveling, for example) and be sure to bring a snack.

FATIGUE OR LACK OF SLEEP

Children who get migraines are especially sensitive to lack of sleep. Other migraine sufferers who are awakened early in the morning, particularly by a bright light (sun shining through an uncovered window), often experience a migraine. People who must change time shifts for their jobs often experience migraines during the adjustment period. Whenever possible, be consistent with your sleep habits.

HORMONAL FACTORS

Menstruation, especially, but also birth control pills, pregnancy, menopause, and estrogen supplements often play a crucial role in triggering migraines in women. Menstrual migraines often are the most severe and tend to be the most difficult to treat. Headaches are usually better during pregnancy, at least in the last two trimesters. (See Chapter 7 for detailed information on the relationship between hormones and migraines in women.)

OVERSLEEPING AND EXCESSIVE SLEEP

Although most children and adolescents are unaffected by oversleeping, too much sleep in adults can lead to a migraine attack. Be careful about regulating your sleep, especially on weekends. Naps can also be a problem. Even just a half hour of extra sleep on a Sunday morning, after a stressful week, may be enough to trigger a migraine.

EXERTION, EXERCISE, OR SEX

For some people, certain types of exertion, including sex, consistently trigger a migraine. Anti-inflammatories taken before exercising or having sex often prevent the headache. (See Chapter 12 for more on exertion and sex headaches.)

BRIGHT LIGHTS

If you get migraines, chances are you are sensitive to bright fluorescent light and sunlight, even when you don't have a headache. Wearing sunglasses can help; be sure to keep a spare pair in the car because windshield glare is a common trigger. Many migraine sufferers are also bothered by oncoming headlights at night. Camera flashes, fluorescent lights in grocery stores, and too much time in front of a computer screen are also triggers.

HEAD TRAUMA

A blow to the head can cause migraines whether or not you have a history of migraine headaches. Rear-end whiplash accidents are common triggers, and the related migraines may persist for months or years. (See Chapter 12 for more on post-traumatic headaches.)

ALTITUDE

Some people get migraines at high altitudes. One reason may be that there is less oxygen high up, and the blood vessels in the body try to compensate by dilating, a cause of headache in some people. Exercise may help by getting more oxygen into the blood. Vitamin C might also help ward off the effects of high altitudes. Sometimes special medications, such as a water pill called Diamox or steroids, can help too.

MOTION

Sometimes travel by car, plane, train, or boat can trigger a migraine for reasons that researchers can't explain. Some children who get motion sickness develop migraines several years later. Preventing motion sickness by riding in the front seat and making frequent road stops may help ward off a potential migraine.

PREVENTING MIGRAINES WITH MEDICATIONS

If you suffer from frequent headaches and the strategies discussed so far are not adequate to relieve them, your doctor may recommend preventive medications, though the ultimate decision to try them will be yours. Think about the fact, however, that you will probably end up taking less medication for migraine prevention than if you simply chase after frequent headaches with pain relievers.

Consider preventive medication if:

1. You get moderate to severe migraines more than three times a month.
2. The medications to relieve the migraines fail to provide adequate relief.
3. Your quality of life is sufficiently compromised by migraine severity or frequency.

4. You are willing to take medication daily, accept that possible side effects may occur, and change medications if necessary.

Although these medications won't usually completely eliminate migraines, they usually significantly reduce the overall impact that migraines have on your life. A trial course of about four weeks is necessary before you can assess a medication's usefulness.

Choosing a preventive medication will depend on factors such as whether you also get chronic tension headaches, your age, sensitivity to side effects, sleeping patterns, stomach sensitivity, blood pressure, pulse, and other medical concerns.

Starting on preventive medication will take some patience and perseverance. Here are some general guidelines:

UNDERSTAND THE GOAL
Although it would be great if you could eliminate 90 to 100 percent of your migraines, that would probably require too much medication with too many side effects. Your goal for reducing migraine frequency, therefore, must be modified to a realistic 50 to 90 percent improvement; your goal for reducing the intensity or severity of your migraines should be a realistic 70 percent improvement.

BE WILLING TO CHANGE
Be open to changing medications if one doesn't work or causes too many side effects. And remember that what worked for someone else won't necessarily work for you.

BE TOLERANT
Try to be willing to endure mildly annoying side effects in order to achieve positive results with the headaches.

BE PATIENT

Many of the medications need several weeks to become fully effective, and doses may need be adjusted. Call your doctor if you have problems or concerns, but try to stick with each medication for the desired length of time.

BE WELL INFORMED

Most of these medications are used for other health conditions besides headache. Learn what they are and why you are using the drug for headache. Be aware of possible side effects so you are not frightened or confused if they occur.

FIRST-LINE MEDICATIONS FOR PREVENTING MIGRAINES

1. ANTIDEPRESSANTS

Although these medications are commonly used at high doses to combat depression, that's not why they are recommended here. Some of these drugs, such as amitriptyline and other similar so-called tricyclic antidepressants, are useful because they tend to increase the concentration of serotonin in the brain. Newer antidepressants, which are not tricyclics, like Prozac, Zoloft, and Paxil also influence serotonin.

Note: Many of these medications can influence heart rate, increasing the risk of a rapid heartbeat. For that reason, they are prescribed with caution for the elderly and are sometimes used with a beta-blocker (the next group of drugs we'll discuss) to lower the pulse.

- **AMITRIPTYLINE (ELAVIL)**

  This is the most commonly prescribed antidepressant because it is effective, inexpensive, and can help you sleep. It is particularly useful if you get both daily tension headaches and migraines.

TYPICAL DOSE: It is important to begin with only 10 mg, which may be all many people can tolerate, taken at night, working up to 25 or 50 mg (doses far below those used to treat depression) in several weeks. The dose can be pushed up to 150 or 200 mg if needed. Some people do well with as little as 5 mg (half a tablet).

SIDE EFFECTS: Sedation (which decreases over time), weight gain, a dry mouth (which can be countered with Oral Balance Gel or Biotene toothpaste), constipation, dizziness. Occasional anxiety or nervousness, which will usually decrease in time. Less common side effects are depression, blurred vision, memory difficulties, and insomnia (although usually amitriptyline induces sleepiness).

- **FLUOXETINE (PROZAC)**

Prozac has fewer side effects than amitriptyline but is expensive. It is extremely effective when depression, anxiety, or panic attacks also occur or if chronic daily headaches are a problem. Although it is a relatively new medication and doctors have only limited experience prescribing it for migraines, so far the results are very promising. Fears about Prozac's link to suicidal or violent thoughts have been disproved.

TYPICAL DOSE: 10 mg (half a capsule) to start in the morning, perhaps raised to 20 mg daily after four days (though 10 mg a day or even every other day is sometimes adequate). To take a half capsule, open the capsule into a cup of juice, drink half the juice, and save the remainder for the next dose. Liquid Prozac also available.

SIDE EFFECTS: Nausea, anxiety or agitation, insomnia. Fatigue, weight gain, or sedation occur much less often with Prozac than with similar drugs. Weight loss and decreased appetite may occur, particularly if you take more than three capsules a day (although some experience this side effect with as little as one capsule). Several side effects are common.

- **DOXEPIN (SINEQUAN)**
Very similar to amitriptyline, doxepin is extremely helpful for migraines and tension headaches, as well as anxiety.

TYPICAL DOSE: Usually begins with only 10 mg, to be taken at night, which is all that many people can tolerate; if tolerated, the dose may be slowly increased to 50 or 75 mg and up to 150 mg or more, but if 150 mg is not effective, the medication should probably be changed. A typical dose is 50 mg.

SIDE EFFECTS: Sedation, weight gain, a dry mouth, dizziness, and constipation. (See side effects for amitriptyline for more detail.)

If the side effects of amitriptyline, fluoxetine, or doxepin are too severe for you, your doctor may recommend one of the following antidepressants. They are only mildly effective for migraine but are quite useful for chronic daily headache.

- **NORTRIPTYLINE (PAMELOR, AVENTYL)**
When amitriptyline has been effective, but its side effects are too severe, doctors sometimes recommend nortriptyline because it causes less sedation; however, it is less effective and more expensive than amitriptyline. Nortriptyline is safer for the elderly than amitriptyline and the other older antidepressants because it has a relatively low risk of cardiac side effects. The new antidepressants, such as Prozac, however, may be even safer. Nortriptyline is also useful for children and adolescents.

TYPICAL DOSE: 10 mg to start, slowly increasing to 25 mg, sometimes to 100 mg, taken at night. Only available as capsules.

SIDE EFFECTS: Similar to amitriptyline but less severe, including sedation (which decreases over time), weight gain, a dry mouth, constipation, or dizziness. Occasional anxiety or nervousness, but these side effects will quickly decrease. Less common side effects are depression, blurred vision, memory difficulties, and insomnia.

- **PROTRIPTYLINE (VIVACTIL)**

Protriptyline is often used when tension headaches are also a problem, or when nortriptyline's side effects, such as sedation and weight gain, are too severe. It is not sedating and does not cause weight gain.

TYPICAL DOSE: 2.5 mg to start each morning, increasing to 5 or 10 mg (sometimes even 30 or 50 mg, the typical doses prescribed for depression).

SIDE EFFECTS: Nervousness. A dry mouth, constipation, and dizziness, though less severe than with nortriptyline may occur. Insomnia (countered by taking it in the morning) occurs often, blurred vision and stomach upset less often.

- **SERTRALINE (ZOLOFT), PAROXETINE (PAXIL)**

Similar to Prozac, Zoloft and Paxil are newer medications that are very well tolerated by most people, though expensive (100-mg tablets of Zoloft are less expensive than two 50-mg tablets). Experience with Zoloft and Paxil and migraines has so far been promising.

TYPICAL DOSE: Zoloft: 25 mg to start, increasing to 50 mg in four days; dose may go as high as 200 mg (the same range that is effective for depression). To be taken once a day, either in the morning or evening. Paxil: 20-mg tablet once a day.

SIDE EFFECTS: Less dryness of the mouth and constipation than with the older antidepressants. May also cause nausea, diarrhea, headache, fatigue, dizziness, tremor, insomnia, sexual dysfunction, or sweating in less than one-quarter of the people who take either drug. Do not usually cause weight gain or sedation, although they may occur.

- **DESIPRAMINE (NORPRAMIN)**

Milder than other antidepressants, desipramine is useful if you are very sensitive to drug side effects. This medication is much more helpful, however, for chronic daily headaches than for migraines (see Chapter 9).

• **TRIMIPRAMINE (SURMONTIL)**

Trimipramine is a good choice when amitriptyline no longer works or if its side effects are too severe. Though well tolerated compared to the other antidepressants, it is sedating. It is usually much more helpful for daily headaches than for migraines (see Chapter 9).

There are other antidepressants, known as MAO inhibitor antidepressants, such as phenelzine (Nardil), which are extremely effective, but their side effects, especially insomnia and weight gain, are severe compared with other antidepressants. Also, if you take an MAO inhibitor antidepressant, you will have to observe a very strict diet for safety reasons.

THE ANTIDEPRESSANTS: COMPARING SIDE EFFECTS

Drug Generic (Trade Name)	Sedation	Weight Gain	Anticholinergic Effect *
Doxepin (Sinequan)	Severe	Severe	Moderate
Amitriptyline (Elavil)	Severe	Severe	Severe
Protriptyline (Vivactil)	None	None	Severe
Fluoxetine (Prozac)	Mild	Mild	None
Sertraline (Zoloft), Paroxetine (Paxil)	Mild	Mild	None
Nortriptyline (Pamelor, Aventyl)	Moderate	Moderate	Moderate
Desipramine (Norpramin)	Mild	Mild	Mild
Trimipramine (Surmontil)	Severe	Severe	Moderate

| Phenelzine (Nardil) | Mild | Very severe | Moderate |

* Tendency of the medication to cause a dry mouth, constipation, difficulty urinating, heartbeat irregularities, sweating, drowsiness, dizziness, and low blood pressure upon standing up suddenly. With the exception of a dry mouth and constipation, other symptoms are relatively rare.

2. BETA-BLOCKERS

Beta-blockers, which prevent blood vessel dilation, are just as effective as amitriptyline in preventing migraines, and in combination with amitriptyline, form the backbone of migraine prevention. Because they lower the pulse (which often gives people the sense of being slowed down), they are often prescribed with amitriptyline (or another antidepressant) to counter the antidepressant's influence in increasing the heart rate.

If you have high blood pressure, taking a beta-blocker can help both the hypertension and the migraines. Beta-blockers also tend to help counter anxiety, but they may contribute to weight gain, depression, fatigue, higher cholesterol levels, diminished interest in sex, and problems concentrating. The side effects cease once you stop taking the drug.

If one beta-blocker doesn't help, your doctor is likely to recommend another because the mechanism of action of the various beta-blockers works differently.

• PROPRANOLOL (INDERAL)

Inderal is by far the most widely studied and most frequently prescribed beta-blocker. It prevents blood vessel dilation and helps stabilize blood flow through a serotonin mechanism. Inderal is often prescribed with amitriptyline for optimal results.

Inderal is usually not recommended if you have asthma or congestive heart failure, and should be used with caution if you have Raynaud's syndrome, a circulatory disorder.

TYPICAL DOSE: 60 mg to start, usually maintained between 60 mg and 160 mg per day. Must taper off to discontinue (except when used in a low dose by a young person, under age thirty, for a short time). Usually, it is taken once a day, in long-acting capsule form.

SIDE EFFECTS: Because propranolol easily enters the central nervous system, side effects such as fatigue are relatively common. Diarrhea, gas, and stomach upset are also fairly common; insomnia, depression, lightheadedness, and difficulty concentrating are less common. Other possible side effects include lethargy, weight gain, less tolerance to exercising, wheezing, and shortness of breath.

- **METOPROLOL (LOPRESSOR)**

This medication occasionally works when propranolol does not. If you get chronic daily headaches as well as migraines, metoprolol may be a good choice.

TYPICAL DOSE: 25 mg to start, twice a day. This may be increased to 50 mg, twice a day. Increasing the dose gradually minimizes side effects.

SIDE EFFECTS: Same as propranolol but with fewer respiratory problems.

- **NADOLOL (CORGARD)**

Nadolol is as effective as propranolol and may work when propranolol does not.

TYPICAL DOSE: 20 mg, increased to 40 through 120 mg, per day, with most people maintaining at 80 mg and lower. The scored tablets make dosage adjustments easy.

SIDE EFFECTS: Similar to propranolol with less fatigue.

- **ATENOLOL (TENORMIN)**

Because this medication doesn't affect the lungs as much as the other beta-blockers do, this medication causes fewer breathing problems. If you have any tendency toward asthma, however, you should use atenolol only with extreme caution.

TYPICAL DOSE: 50 mg, once a day. This may be increased to 100 mg per day, if necessary.

SIDE EFFECTS: Possibly less sedation and less fatigue than with propranolol.

- **TIMOLOL (BLOCADREN)**

Timolol is also sometimes effective when the other beta-blockers have failed.

TYPICAL DOSE: To minimize side effects, this medication is usually started with 5 mg taken twice a day, then up to 20 or 30 mg twice a day, the average daily dose, if necessary.

SIDE EFFECTS: Same as propranolol, but possibly with less sedation.

3. NONSTEROIDAL ANTI-INFLAMMATORIES (NSAIDs)

The NSAIDs can be very effective for preventing migraines, but their use is limited because they tend to cause gastrointestinal distress (stomach upset or ulcers) and potentially serious liver and kidney irritation. That's why amitriptyline (or perhaps another antidepressant) and a beta-blocker are usually chosen first.

But for women under age forty suffering from menstrual migraines (and menstrual cramps), and for those who are under age forty and very sensitive to the sedating effects of the beta-blockers and antidepressants, NSAIDs may be a good choice, although they are relatively expensive. They also can help with arthritis or musculoskeletal problems (painful knee, back, shoulder).

If you have found NSAIDs effective as an abortive medication (to dull the pain of a migraine in progress) and your doctor recommends switching to a daily preventive medication, a lower-dose NSAID may be right for you because you know it works and that you are tolerant of its potential side effects. Remember, however, always to take these medications with food.

- **NAPROXEN (ALEVE, NAPROSYN, ANAPROX)**

Naproxen is the most widely studied and most frequently prescribed NSAID for migraines, but it is recommended only if you are under age fifty. It can be particularly useful if you get menstrual migraines and daily headaches. Naproxen is sometimes combined with another first-line preventive medication (such as amitriptyline) to enhance effectiveness.

TYPICAL DOSE: 500 or 550 mg once a day, sometimes twice a day. An over-the-counter version, Aleve, is available in a lower dosage, 200 mg per tablet.

SIDE EFFECTS: The most common is stomach upset. If you find that naproxen is very effective for your migraines but gives you an upset stomach, your doctor may recommend using a sucralfate (Carafate) pill taken with liquid half an hour or an hour before taking the naproxen; alternatively, cimetidine (Tagamet) can usually prevent an upset stomach.

Other potential side effects include skin rashes, fatigue, fluid retention (swelling of hands or feet), ringing in the ear, and tension headaches. When used chronically, the liver and kidneys need to be periodically monitored with a simple blood test.

- **FENOPROFEN (NALFON)**

Fenoprofen is useful when naproxen can't be tolerated or is ineffective; it is sometimes useful for daily headaches.

TYPICAL DOSE: 600 mg a day to start, increased up to two or three times a day. 200 mg doses are sometimes used to prevent migraines in children.

SIDE EFFECTS: Risk of kidney and liver irritation; must be monitored periodically with blood tests.

- **FLURBIPROFEN (ANSAID)**

Well tolerated, flurbiprofen is particularly useful for menstrual headaches (see Chapter 7).

TYPICAL DOSE: 100 mg twice a day.

SIDE EFFECTS: Same as with fenoprofen.

- **KETOPROFEN (ORUDIS)**

Ketoprofen is quite helpful in preventing migraines, and sometimes tension headaches.

TYPICAL DOSE: 75 mg to 150 mg per day. Now available as a very convenient once-a-day 200-mg preparation called Oruvail.

SIDE EFFECTS: Similar to the other NSAIDs; liver and kidney should be regularly monitored.

4. CALCIUM BLOCKERS

A relatively new treatment for preventing migraines, calcium blockers are generally not as effective as antidepressants or beta-blockers. However, they have far fewer side effects and do not usually cause the weight gain or lethargy that these other preventive medications often do. If you are an athlete or would be particularly dismayed by a beta-blocker's effect of impeding athletic performance, you may want to ask your doctor about using calcium blockers to prevent your migraines.

The primary medication prescribed in this group is verapamil, although nifedipine (Procardia) and diltiazem (Cardizem) are occasionally helpful.

- **VERAPAMIL (ISOPTIN, CALAN, VERELAN)**

  This is the most widely prescribed and most effective calcium blocker, but it may take up to six weeks to become effective. Also useful for cluster and chronic daily headaches, verapamil is often combined with amitriptyline or naproxen to maximize relief. If you have Raynaud's syndrome, a circulatory disorder common among migraine sufferers, then verapamil may be a particularly good choice for you as it helps counteract the problems associated with Raynaud's.

  TYPICAL DOSE: Convenient once-a-day tablet, 120 mg to start, increased to an average of 180 or 240 a day.

  SIDE EFFECTS: Relatively few other than constipation, which is very common. Occasional skin rashes, dizziness, insomnia, swelling of hands and feet, and anxiety. Fatigue is less common.

SECOND-LINE MEDICATIONS FOR PREVENTING MIGRAINES

1. TWO FIRST-LINE PREVENTIVE MEDICATIONS

In some cases, using two medications can be effective when each medication used individually was not. Typically, a doctor may suggest combining two preventive medications if you:

- **HAVE TRIED INDIVIDUAL MEDICATIONS, BUT THEY HAVEN'T WORKED.**
  Usually doctors prescribe one preventive medication at a time, starting with low doses and raising them slowly if needed. Most people appreciate this approach, are prepared to wait for the medications to work, and are willing to switch medications if necessary.

- **ARE EXTREMELY FRUSTRATED AND WANT FAST RESULTS.**
  When you have moderate or severe chronic daily headaches as well as bothersome migraines, you and your doctor may decide to push ahead at a faster rate with the preventive approach. Depending on how severe your headaches are and how frustrated you are with treatments, your doctor has several ways he can try to accelerate your treatment, among them increasing your doses more quickly than usual.

- **ARE SUFFERING FROM A NEW ONSET OF SEVERE HEADACHES.**
  If you have become very upset and frustrated with head pain because your headaches seem to be worsening or becoming more frequent, the doctor may decide to push preventive medication at a faster pace.

Typically, the doses and potential side effects of using two medications together are the same as when they are used individually. Here are some common pairings that doctors use to prevent migraines.

- **AMITRIPTYLINE WITH PROPRANOLOL**
  When amitriptyline increases heart rate, propranolol is often added to neutralize the effect. This combination is often used when both migraines and chronic daily headaches are problems.

- **NSAID WITH ANOTHER FIRST-LINE MEDICATION**
  Naproxen (or another NSAID) is often prescribed with amitriptyline (an antidepressant), propranolol (a beta-blocker), or verapamil (a calcium blocker) to serve as both preventive and abortive medications.

If you are over fifty, however, an NSAID is usually a third-line choice because of the increased risk of gastrointestinal, kidney, and liver problems.

• **PROPRANOLOL AND VERAPAMIL**

These two medications are occasionally combined in small doses when they have not been effective individually. However, heart and blood pressure need to be monitored in these cases.

2. METHYSERGIDE (SANSERT)

This extremely powerful preventive medication seems to help constrict swollen blood vessels and affect serotonin, but it is not commonly used because of the possible side effect of fibrosis, a "thickening" about the lungs, heart, or kidneys which occurs in one out of seven hundred patients. With careful use and low doses, however, it can be relatively safe and effective.

Methysergide is most often prescribed for people forty-five and younger because its constricting effect on blood vessels can present a problem in older people. It is also not a good choice if you have coronary artery disease, previous blood clots (thrombophlebitis), peptic ulcers, kidney or liver problems, or any vascular disorders. If you have high blood pressure, your doctor should closely monitor you on this medication.

TYPICAL DOSE: 2 mg to start, working up to an average dose of 2 mg twice a day, taken with food. Taking a one-month rest from the medication after six months is often recommended, though controversial, to try to prevent fibrosis. A substitute medication can be prescribed during that time.

SIDE EFFECTS: Nausea, hot feelings in the head, and leg cramps are common. Occasional severe gastrointestinal upset. "Feeling weird" is not unusual, although most people do not have significant side effects with methysergide.

3. VALPROATE (DEPAKOTE)

This is a very useful medication when migraines have not responded to the more common treatments. If you have liver problems, however, it is not a good choice.

TYPICAL DOSE: 250 mg per day, to start, with food, increased over two weeks to an average dose of 500 mg once or twice a day (sometimes up to 2,500 a day), usually limited by side effects. It takes at least four weeks to know if the drug works well.

SIDE EFFECTS: Nausea, stomach upset, and sedation. With higher doses, you may be hungrier and gain weight. Less common side effects include mild impairment in cognitive skills, hair loss (usually temporary), tremors (in which case the dose should be lowered and then discontinued if the condition persists), lethargy, mood swings, and fatigue.

THIRD-LINE MEDICATIONS FOR
PREVENTING MIGRAINES

These third-line approaches to preventing migraines are usually the treatment of last resort. Doctors won't prescribe them until you have tried other options that have potentially fewer problems. Although all these treatments are used with caution, your doctor will take even greater precautions if you are over fifty.

1. MAO (MONOAMINE OXIDASE) INHIBITORS
These medications are helpful if you get severe migraines (or chronic daily headaches) and other medications haven't worked. They also can be very helpful to counter depression, anxiety, and panic attacks.

Although MAO inhibitors may be used with relative safety and may be the only medications that will help prevent your migraines and daily headaches, it is essential that you avoid certain foods and medications while taking an MAO inhibitor because they could significantly increase the risk of a high blood pressure crisis:

- Sumatriptan (Imitrex)
- Meperidine (Demerol)
- Over-the-counter decongestants (Check with the doctor if you want to take any OTC medication.)
- Excessive caffeine (more than two cups of coffee or cola drinks), chocolate
- Red wine, sherry, ale, and beer
- Tenderized meats, liver, fermented meats (pepperoni, summer sausage, salami, bologna)
- Caviar, dried or salted fish, herring
- Aged cheeses
- Yogurt, sour cream
- Bananas, overripe figs, avocado, raisins
- Yeast extracts, soy sauce
- Fava beans

Occasionally, an MAO inhibitor is used in conjunction with certain other antidepressants, beta-blockers, and calcium blockers; if you take such a combination, your doctor will need to monitor you closely.

- **PHENELZINE (NARDIL)**

This is the most effective and frequently used MAO inhibitor, but liver function and blood pressure need be monitored with its use.

TYPICAL DOSE: 15 mg to start, taken at night, and sometimes increased over one to three weeks to an average dose of 45 mg if needed. If ineffective even at 75 mg, then another medication should be tried instead. Take at night to avoid interactions with certain foods. If phenelzine causes insomnia, try taking it in the early morning.

SIDE EFFECTS: Insomnia and weight gain. Less common side effects include a dry mouth, constipation, rapid heartbeat, agitation or other mood changes, swelling of the hands or feet.

2. MAO INHIBITOR WITH A FIRST-LINE PREVENTIVE MEDICATION

Sometimes an MAO inhibitor, commonly phenelzine (Nardil), is combined with a calcium blocker or an antidepressant with the hope that using two preventive medications will work.

- **PHENELZINE (NARDIL) WITH THE CALCIUM BLOCKER VERAPAMIL (ISOPTIN, CALAN, VERELAN)**

   This powerful combination may help severe migraines that haven't responded to other drugs. Verapamil relieves pain and neutralizes the high blood pressure risk. Nevertheless, your blood pressure should be monitored if you use this combination.

   TYPICAL DOSE: 30 to 60 mg per day of Nardil, with 120 to 240 of verapamil, starting with low doses and gradually increasing over two weeks with frequent blood pressure checks.

   SIDE EFFECTS: Same as with phenelzine alone.

3. INTRAVENOUS DIHYDROERGOTAMINE (IV DHE)

This treatment is very safe and extremely effective for preventing and relieving frequent or severe migraines, daily headaches, or cluster headaches, but its use requires going to a doctor's office or hospital to receive intravenous injections. Typically, IV DHE will give you good relief for at least one or two months, occasionally for as long as eight months.

Your doctor may also recommend this treatment if you have become dependent on narcotic painkillers, such as codeine, or analgesic overuse, and, as a result, you suffer from rebound headaches. This medication can help you withdraw from your dependence.

If you have high blood pressure, your doctor will treat you cautiously with the medication. If you have heart disease or peripheral vascular disease, your doctor probably won't use it at all.

TYPICAL DOSE: *When administered at the doctor's office,* the doctor will ask you take an antinausea medication at home, preferably Reglan because it is mild, and a few Tums. At the office, you will get an injection, probably a shot twice a day for one to three days, or a total of two to six doses.

When administered at the hospital, the injection can be given three times in one day, or up to nine doses in three days. The accompanying antinausea medication can be stronger, so you can take larger doses, which, in turn, will be more sedating. Typically, you'll need a two- or three-day stay in the hospital, so the staff can monitor and care for you.

SIDE EFFECTS: Nausea, hot feeling in the head, a temporary tightness in the throat or chest, leg and muscle cramps, and a temporary rise in blood pressure. Occasional diarrhea or brief muscle tension headache afterward. The side effects, if present, usually last less than one hour. To combat nausea, which is common, an antinausea medication is usually taken before the DHE.

NEW APPROACHES

Stimulants (Ritalin) or long-acting narcotics (methadone) are occasionally used if other methods have not been effective.

CASE STUDY

Here is an example of how this preventive information might be applied in a real situation.

MIMI

INITIAL VISIT: Mimi, a twenty-two-year-old news service writer, gets about one migraine every week. Her migraines started at age fourteen but have increased in the past year. Mimi has asthma, but otherwise is healthy.

She tends to get more migraines around her menstrual period

and with stress or weather changes. Red wine also gives her a migraine. Mimi gets some relief from Excedrin or Fiorinal, but the headaches are severe, with nausea accompanying most of them. Mimi's mom also gets migraines.

With four severe migraines a month, Mimi is on the borderline between needing daily preventive medication and treating the headaches once they begin. She is placed on naproxen, a nonsteroidal anti-inflammatory, once a day as a preventive medication. The NSAIDs have an advantage because they do not cause drowsiness or weight gain; however, they can irritate the stomach, liver, or kidneys. Mimi is also taught to inject sumatriptan (Imitrex), which is expensive but very effective in relieving migraines in progress.

WEEK 6: The migraines are down to two per month and the Imitrex works well, stopping the headache within one hour.

WEEK 12: By this time, both medications seem to be losing their effectiveness. So Mimi's doctor changes her daily preventive from naproxen to verapamil (Isoptin, Calan, Verelan), which does not affect Mimi's asthma (a beta-blocker, such as Inderal, would affect the asthma). And the sumatriptan is changed to Midrin, to relieve a migraine when it occurs. The doctor tells her she can take up to five capsules of Midrin in one day, and also gives her Compazine capsules for nausea.

WEEK 16: The verapamil is ineffective. Mimi is getting at least four migraines a month. The Midrin is partially effective, although it makes her feel somewhat lightheaded; the Compazine helps decrease her nausea. Mimi's doctor takes her off the verapamil as a preventive medication and gives her amitriptyline, an antidepressant that is widely used to prevent headaches.

WEEK 20: Mimi sleeps well with the amitriptyline because of its sedative effect, but the doses are kept low and she does not have a problem with daytime drowsiness. The headaches are down to one per month. Although the Midrin is somewhat effective to relieve a migraine when it occurs, Mimi also begins taking Fiorinal, either alone or with the Midrin, to enhance pain relief.

THE FUTURE: As her condition and sensitivity to side effects shifts, Mimi's medication may change. Her doctor may take her off preventives altogether, or switch her to another preventive, perhaps a different NSAID or antidepressant. There are also other abortives that may be more effective, such as ergotamines, DHE nasal spray or injection, or Norgesic Forte.

7

WOMEN, HORMONES, AND MIGRAINES

FLUCTUATING HORMONES, especially the progestins and estrogens, seem to play an important role in influencing migraines in women. At age ten, as many boys as girls suffer from migraines. By puberty, many girls who never before had migraine problems start having them, and by the midteens, migraines become much more common and more severe among girls than boys.

Puberty and the days around ovulation and menstruation are particularly vulnerable times for women who are susceptible to migraines. A woman's thirties and forties are commonly the worst decades, with the migraines becoming severe and prolonged. Most women experience relief during pregnancy and often after menopause. Birth control pills occasionally trigger, yet occasionally improve migraines, but for most women they don't exert much influence on the pattern of headaches.

Researchers aren't sure exactly why women's hormones affect migraines. One theory is that the hormones influence the mechanisms underlying migraines. Another theory is that a sex-linked chromosome may be involved. As we've already discussed, most migraines are inherited.

MENSTRUAL MIGRAINES

Menstrual migraines can be especially miserable because they're often more severe and harder to treat than other kinds of migraines. Typically, they occur before, during, or after a woman's period. If you suffer from menstrual migraines, you may have headaches during ovulation and get migraines that aren't triggered by hormones at other times of the month as well.

HORMONAL INFLUENCES

Researchers suspect that the hormone mechanisms, which are controlled by the brain, are somehow different in women who get hormonal, or menstrual, headaches than in other women, though consistent patterns haven't emerged. Some studies have found that women who get premenstrual migraines have higher levels of the hormones progestin and estrogen before their periods than women who don't get headaches. Others suggest that a drop in estrogen levels, which occurs just before a period (and after menopause or a hysterectomy), can trigger headaches (yet in other women this drop helps their migraines). Still other menstrual migraines may be related to the fluid build-up that occurs with menstruation.

Both estrogen and the progestin progesterone are known to influence serotonin receptors, and low levels of estrogen can significantly impact the hypothalamus (the gland that controls the hormonal secretion functions) and its control mechanisms. The truth is, researchers do not yet understand the mechanisms behind hormones and headaches.

TREATING MENSTRUAL MIGRAINES

Mild to moderate menstrual headaches that last only a day or so can often be relieved with one of the over-the-counter medications or anti-inflammatories discussed in Chapter 2, such as Excedrin, ibuprofen, or a prescription NSAID.

Severe, prolonged menstrual migraines, which are not uncommon, can be relieved with injections and then prevented by following several approaches, as summarized below.

RELIEVING MENSTRUAL MIGRAINES: In general, your doctor will probably use the same strategies to relieve a menstrual migraine as a general migraine. When the migraines are severe, the cortisone medications, especially Decadron or Prednisone, are among the most effective treatments. Injections of DHE, ketorolac, or sumatriptan are also powerful treatments for severe menstrual migraines. If these strategies fail, a strong narcotic taken with a strong antinausea medication, such as chlorpromazine (Thorazine) can help. Because menstrual migraines can be severe, many women must resort to these powerful treatments. Refer to Chapter 5 for detailed discussions of these medications.

PREVENTING MENSTRUAL MIGRAINES: As with general migraines, your menstrual migraines may be triggered by typical migraine foods, as outlined in Chapter 6. However, you may be sensitive to these foods only the week or so before your periods. To prevent menstrual migraines, experiment with abstaining from alcohol (especially red wine), chocolate, aged cheese, and other common migraine-trigger foods; eating regularly and including plenty of complex carbohydrates (pasta, rice, beans, whole grains) to maintain steady levels of blood sugar; exercising; and using relaxation techniques to minimize stress. Also experiment with caffeine — in some women, caffeine helps; in others, it is a trigger. Some doctors will also recommend supplements of vitamin B_6 (100 mg a day) and vitamin E (400 IU a day).

If your menstrual migraines are predictable, moderately severe, and not responsive to nonmedication strategies, your doctor may suggest trying preventive medication beginning on the day before the expected onset of the migraine and continuing until two to three days past the time you normally get migraines. Details on medications doctors typically use for preventing menstrual migraines follow. *Note: Many of the medications mentioned in this chapter have been discussed in detail in previous chapters. Please check the index to locate more detailed information.*

MEDICATIONS FOR TREATING
MENSTRUAL MIGRAINES

1. NONSTEROIDAL ANTI-INFLAMMATORIES (NSAIDS) (NAPROXEN, IBUPROFEN, FLURBIPROFEN)

Anti-inflammatories are the backbone of preventive therapy for menstrual migraines because they have the fewest side effects and are well tolerated. When one NSAID doesn't work, your doctor will probably suggest trying another before progressing to a different class of medications.

TYPICAL DOSE: Take three days before expected headache and continue until several days past the expected time. Timing can be tricky. For ibuprofen, from 400 mg to 2,400 mg per day, split up during day. For naproxen, 500 mg, once or twice a day. For flurbiprofen (Ansaid), 100 mg twice a day.

SIDE EFFECTS: Stomach upset.

2. ERGOTAMINE DERIVATIVES

These medications are often effective, although they do carry a risk for triggering rebound headaches.

- **ERGOTAMINE TARTRATE**

  TYPICAL DOSE: Usually 2 mg of ergotamine per day.

  SIDE EFFECTS: In addition to rebound headaches, ergotamine derivatives may cause nausea or severe gastrointestinal upset, as well as nervousness and leg cramps.

- **BELLERGAL-S**

  This medication also contains an antinausea medication and a barbiturate sedative. Because it is sedating, it is usually taken the night before the expected headache and continued for several days.

TYPICAL DOSE: One to two tablets each night.

SIDE EFFECTS: Sedation.

- **ERGONOVINE (ERGOTRATE)**

This medication is well tolerated and occasionally effective.

TYPICAL DOSE: 0.2 mg, two to four times a day.

SIDE EFFECTS: Same as the other ergotamines, though usually milder.

- **DIHYDROERGOTAMINE (DHE)**

This medication must be either injected, made into suppositories by a pharmacist, or taken as a new nasal spray that is very convenient. DHE is usually very well tolerated.

TYPICAL DOSE: 1 mg a day.

SIDE EFFECTS: Nausea, harmless throat or chest tightness, mild muscle contraction, headache, leg cramps, a hot feeling about the head.

- **METHYSERGIDE (SANSERT)**

Although this medication is powerful and very effective, it sometimes causes severe side effects, though they'll usually stop within a few hours.

TYPICAL DOSE: 2 mg once a day with food; may be increased up to three or four pills a day.

SIDE EFFECTS: Gastrointestinal upset, nausea, leg cramps. Many people also experience a flushed and hot feeling about the head. Dizziness or lightheadedness may be extreme.

3. DIURETICS

DYAZIDE, HYDROCHLOROTHIAZIDE, AND MODURETIC

Diuretics, also known as water pills, are occasionally helpful for migraines and also help other menstrual symptoms, such as bloating. They are generally well tolerated, but even though they are used for only a short time during the month, care must be taken to avoid losing too much potassium. Diuretics should be taken only under a doctor's care.

TYPICAL DOSE: Half a pill or one pill taken in the morning for two to three days prior to and with the menstrual period.

SIDE EFFECTS: Frequent urination. Occasional rashes, weakness, or dizziness.

4. HORMONAL APPROACHES

If NSAIDs, ergotamines, and diuretics don't work, and your menstrual migraines are very severe and debilitating, your doctor may recommend a stronger approach, such as hormonal therapy. Before trying these powerful drugs, though, be sure you are well informed of the potential risks. They often have unpleasant side effects, which you'll have to weigh against the pain and degraded quality of life you suffer from headaches.

• TAMOXIFEN (NOLVADEX)

One of the more effective menstrual migraine preventives, this medication is otherwise used in breast cancer therapy. It sometimes decreases the frequency and severity of migraines and daily headaches that occur at other times of the month as well.

TYPICAL DOSE: 10 mg (the range is 5 mg to 20 mg) each day for seven to fourteen days, starting just before menstruation, sometimes earlier.

SIDE EFFECTS: Occasional and mild nausea, hot flashes, and menstrual irregularities; infrequent rashes, vaginal bleeding, vaginal discharges, weight gain, edema, headaches, shortness of breath, loss of appetite, pain in the legs, blurred vision, and dizziness. In very large doses in animals, malignant liver tumors have been reported. Frequent Pap smears are necessary.

• ESTROGEN

If your migraines are severe, prolonged, and generally debilitating, they may warrant using a strong medication. Estrogen sometimes works to prevent menstrual migraines that are triggered by the estrogen decrease that occurs during the late luteal phase of the menstrual cycle. In some women, however, estrogen exacerbates headaches.

TYPICAL DOSE: 0.05 mg of ethinyl estradiol (Estinyl) each day for five days before menses and continued for two days after flow. Or 1 or 2 mg of micronized estradiol (Estrace) each day with same regimen. Or an estrogen skin patch (Estraderm) changed twice weekly and used for a total of seven days.

SIDE EFFECTS: Estrogen carries many potential side effects, including breakthrough bleeding, irregular or suspended periods, menstrual flow changes, endometrial hyperplasia, yeast infection (vaginal candidiasis), nausea, abdominal cramps, colitis or cholestatic jaundice, hair loss (alopecia) or abnormal hair growth (hirsutism), hives, headache, dizziness, depression, weight gain or loss, edema, decreased libido, and tenderness of the breasts. Long-term use may also increase the risk of endometrial cancer and breast cancer.

• **ESTROGEN PLUS METHYLTESTOSTERONE**
Sometimes, a small amount of methyltestosterone (typically used for breast cancer, breast pain, and engorgement after giving birth, among other conditions) improves estrogen therapy.

TYPICAL DOSE: 5 mg each day with the estrogen, usually for seven days.

SIDE EFFECTS: Although uncommon, there are many potential side effects, including menstrual problems, deepening of the voice, excessive hair growth (hirsutism), acne, edema, nausea, cholestatic jaundice, changes in libido, headaches, nervousness, depression, excitation, insomnia, rashes, and alterations in liver function tests.

- **DANAZOL (DANOCRINE)**

Usually used for endometriosis, danazol occasionally prevents menstrual migraines.

TYPICAL DOSE: 200 mg, once a day (and adjusted up or down to 100 to 300 mg per day), starting three to five days prior to the expected time of the headache and continued for three days after it.

SIDE EFFECTS: Although there are many potential side effects, they are usually mild and may include acne, excessive hair growth (hirsutism) or loss (alopecia), edema, sweating and flushing, nervousness, liver problems, weight gain, deepening of the voice, decrease in breast size, vaginitis, emotional swings, rashes, headaches, insomnia, fatigue, changes in libido, and increased blood pressure.

HEADACHES DURING PREGNANCY

If you suffer from migraines, chances are pregnancy, especially the second and third trimesters, will bring a welcome relief. If you do get headaches at this time, however, they are particularly hard to treat because you must avoid drugs that may potentially be harmful to the fetus. First try ice packs, relaxation therapy, rest in a dark room. Ask your doctor about using small amounts of medication, such as acetaminophen (Tylenol). While caffeine decreases headaches, its use during pregnancy remains controversial. If you need something stronger, the doctor may try small doses of meperidine (Demerol), hydrocodone (Vicodin), or acetaminophen with codeine. Take antinausea medications only if absolutely necessary, and only in small amounts.

If your migraines are frequent and severe, or you get daily headaches that are intolerable, your doctor may recommend preventive medications with minimal doses after the first trimester. A beta-blocker (such as propranolol, metoprolol, nadolol, timolol, or atenolol) is often prescribed and discontinued three weeks before delivery to avoid harming the baby. Be sure you understand all the risks before trying any of these medications.

When beta-blockers don't work or can't be used, the doctor may recommend a very low dose (such as 10 or 25 mg) of amitriptyline if daily preventive medication is necessary. However, there have been isolated reports that amitriptyline may trigger abnormalities in babies' arms or legs. Again, be sure you understand whatever risks that this or other medications pose during pregnancy.

MIGRAINES DURING AND AFTER MENOPAUSE

Typically, migraines worsen during menopause, but then may improve afterward. Yet it is not uncommon to have a different experience: Some women get worse headaches after menopause; others enjoy a complete cessation of head pain. Some women who have never had a headache problem get severe migraines for the first time during menopause. Still other women experience no change in their migraine patterns.

If you find yourself getting migraines during menopause, first try the drugless strategies, which can be enormously helpful. If they don't help, your doctor may suggest trying estrogen replacement therapy, estrogen supplements to compensate for diminishing levels of estrogen production. This treatment occasionally improves a migraine problem, although it often causes headaches.

If you get migraines and have been using estrogens and cyclic progestins (progesterone), be sure to discuss your headaches with your doctor immediately. Chances are, the progestins are giving you problems and your doctor will probably discontinue them. Ask about estrogen in a skin patch or injection, as these modes seem to cause fewer problems. Sometimes adding hormones called androgens (methyltestosterone) can help relieve headaches and help counter the side effects of menopause.

CASE STUDY

Here is a fairly typical case of a woman who gets menstrual migraines and how her doctor helps her manage them.

SALLY

INITIAL VISIT: Sally, a thirty-four-year-old teacher and mother of two children, gets severe migraines for four days each month, usually beginning one day before her menstrual period. She has regular periods, every twenty-eight days, and no other health problems. She has tried, with little or no benefit, ibuprofen, Fiorinal, Midrin, Tylenol 3, Vicodin, and Excedrin.

Because Sally usually begins sensing the migraine just prior to the beginning of her period, she is advised to start naproxen, an NSAID, three days before her menstrual period. Naproxen is particularly effective in preventing menstrual migraines. For an abortive medication, the doctor prescribes sumatriptan (Imitrex) tablets because Sally does not want to give herself injections.

FOUR MONTHS LATER: Sally reports that the naproxen helped for the first two months, but then lost its effectiveness. The sumatriptan does not help much, nauseates her, and causes chest heaviness, which she was prepared to expect. Sally's doctor prescribes flurbiprofen (Ansaid), another NSAID, as a preventive medication, ergotamine suppositories (Cafergot), and a small dose of dexamethasone (Decadron) as an abortive medication.

TWO MONTHS LATER: Sally says the flurbiprofen was not effective and because she gets incapacitating and prolonged (four days) migraine attacks, she is prepared to try hormonal therapy to prevent them. She and her doctor discuss fully the risks and possible side effects, from nausea, hot flashes, and rashes to vaginal discharges, weight gain, and shortness of breath. Sally receives a prescription for estrogen to take before her periods to prevent the attacks. Her abortive regimen is working in that it shortens her attacks significantly.

TWO MONTHS LATER: The estrogen is not effective, so Sally's doctor prescribes tamoxifen (Nolvadex) to take for one week before menstrual periods.

TWO MONTHS LATER: Sally reports that the tamoxifen is working well and that she feels in good control. When she does get a migraine, the ergotamine and dexamethasone usually help.

8

TREATING
TENSION HEADACHES
IN PROGRESS

MIGRAINES may be the most common headaches treated by doctors, but tension headaches plague the general population much more commonly; more than three-quarters of all headaches are tension headaches.

WHAT IS A TENSION HEADACHE?

Tension headaches can hurt anywhere around the head, but usually they cause pain on both sides. Sufferers often describe them as band-like, aching, pressing, tightening, or dull. Some people wake up in the early morning with the headache pounding or throbbing. Although usually mild or moderate, these headaches can be severe, waxing and waning throughout the day.

Unlike migraines, these milder headaches come on with no warning or auras, but most people can go on coping with work or home responsibilities. When tension headaches are severe, however, they may be accompanied by dizziness, nausea, and sensitivity to bright lights, much like migraines. Because it is sometimes difficult to distinguish between a severe tension headache and a mild migraine, many researchers suspect that the two headaches are the same illness, with tension headaches at the milder end of the spectrum.

Tension headaches may start at any age; about 40 percent of people start getting them in childhood or in their teens. Whether they will continue for a lifetime is unpredictable. Almost 50 percent of children and adolescents with tension headaches do outgrow their headaches by age twenty. However, if a child has had daily headaches for several years and has a parent who has had migraines or daily headaches, the child is likely to have them for years as well, although they may stop for months or even years, and then recur. In adults who get migraines and tension headaches, the migraines usually decline after age fifty but the tension headache pattern often persists.

TYPES OF TENSION HEADACHES

Usually tension headaches occur periodically and in most cases, an over-the-counter pain reliever, a nap, and a relaxation exercise will relieve them. Ice packs applied to the head may also help.

When they occur more frequently, though, they are either *episodic,* occurring at least twice a week, but not more than fifteen times a month, or *chronic* or *daily,* occurring more than fifteen days a month for at least six months, or almost every day. The lines between the two get blurry if you get spells of daily tension headaches for weeks or months, and then very few headaches for a period of time. Also, many people who get tension headaches get migraines from time to time. For some people, the daily tension headache is much more of a problem than the occasional migraine; other people don't mind the daily headaches but are compelled to do something about their migraines.

TENSION HEADACHES: NOT PSYCHOLOGICAL
BUT INHERITED

Just like migraine headaches, tension headaches are not psychological or "all in the head" but legitimate medical illnesses. Although stress and tension trigger the headaches or make them worse, they are not the true cause of the pain. In fact, the term "tension headache" is erroneous and promotes this misconception. That is why many doctors call these headaches "muscle contraction headaches" instead. As with migraines, the real root of the headache, or cause, is a genetically inherited predisposition to triggers that produce increased muscular tension and changes in blood vessels and the central nervous system. The triggers may be stress, depression, anxiety, or other factors.

Researchers suspect that tension headaches, like migraines, are caused by serotonin changes in the brain. In many ways, tension headaches and migraines are related.

• Both respond to similar medications: antidepressants, calcium blockers, anti-inflammatories, and beta-blockers.
• Both are linked to similar biochemical changes.
• Both are commonly associated with neck pain and muscle spasm.
• Both are often linked to a family history of headaches.
• Both commonly involve muscle tenderness on the head and brain blood flow changes.
• A mild migraine is very difficult to distinguish from a severe tension headache.
• The vast majority of people with chronic daily headaches also get migraines.

TREATMENT FOR TENSION HEADACHES

When the occasional tension headache occurs, the correct way to treat it is very similar to the suggestions offered in Chapter 2.

- Use a relaxation technique.
- Apply ice to your head.
- Try to ignore the pain if it is mild.
- Consider taking medication.

As always, the goal is to take as little medication as possible. If you need medication, your doctor will probably begin by suggesting a first-line abortive. These medications can be very effective, but if overused they carry the risk of causing rebound headaches. If you take numerous pills on a daily basis — more than five a day — you need to use relaxation methods more regularly or consider trying preventive medication.

All these medications are discussed in detail in Chapters 2, 5, and 6. We present them here in order of preference for tension headaches, and review their most salient features.

FIRST-LINE MEDICATIONS FOR
ABORTING TENSION HEADACHES

1. ACETAMINOPHEN

Although less effective than aspirin or the medications that follow, acetaminophen is more easily tolerated. If you take more than 1,500 mg a day on a daily basis, rebound headaches may occur and you should consider daily preventive medication. (See Chapter 2.)

ASPIRIN

Aspirin is more effective than acetaminophen but has a greater risk of side effects. (See Chapter 2.)

2. NAPROXEN (ALEVE)

The OTC version of naproxen is a very effective anti-inflammatory but can commonly cause stomach upset and nausea. (See Chapter 2.)

IBUPROFEN (MOTRIN, ADVIL, NUPRIN, RUFEN, HALTRAN, IBUPRIN, MEDIPREN, MIDOL 200, TRENDAR)

Ibuprofen is also more effective than acetaminophen but may not be more effective than aspirin; stomach upset is relatively common. (See Chapter 2.)

3. CAFFEINE

Taking caffeine, in coffee, soda, or pill form, can be very helpful. It may be taken individually or with a pain reliever to enhance its effectiveness. Caffeine overuse can also lead to rebound headaches. (See Chapter 2.)

4. CAFFEINE-ASPIRIN COMBINATIONS

By combining the effects of caffeine with the pain relief of aspirin, these OTC products, such as Excedrin Extra-Strength or Anacin, can be very effective, but again, avoid overuse. (See Chapter 2.)

5. NAPROXEN (ANAPROX DS)

Higher-dose prescription version naproxen is a very effective anti-inflammatory whose effects may be further enhanced with caffeine. Nausea and stomach upset are common. (See Chapter 5.)

6. FLURBIPROFEN (ANSAID)

A newer prescription anti-inflammatory, flurbiprofen is well tolerated, although stomach upset is common. Used as a preventive for migraines, it can be used as an abortive for tension headaches if the frequency of the 100-mg dose is increased from twice daily to every three or four hours, as needed, but no more than 400 mg per day. (See Chapter 6.)

7. MIDRIN

Midrin, a combination of a blood vessel constrictor, mild non-addicting sedative, and acetaminophen, is effective, safe, and well tolerated. Fatigue and stomach upset are fairly common. By prescription only. (See Chapter 5.)

8. NORGESIC FORTE

Norgesic Forte, a combination of aspirin, caffeine, and a non-addicting muscle relaxant, is one of the strongest nonaddicting abortive medications for tension (and migraine) headaches, but gastrointestinal upset and fatigue are common. (See Chapter 5.)

SECOND-LINE MEDICATIONS FOR
ABORTING TENSION HEADACHES

If the first-line abortives don't work, your doctor may suggest stronger therapy with a more powerful pain reliever. These medications, which are potentially addicting, include the butalbital compounds (first-line migraine abortives), the narcotics (second-line migraine abortives), or the benzodiazepines (also second-line migraine abortives). If you take them once a week or less, these medications don't pose a problem. If you need them almost daily, they can be habit-forming and you should try preventive medication.

In rare circumstances — when first-line abortives, relaxation therapy, and preventive medications fail or cause too many side effects, and you and your doctor are confident that you would never use the medication to get high or lift you out of the dumps — your doctor may suggest using limited amounts of these habit-forming medications on a daily basis. We discuss all of these medications in more detail in Chapter 5, and we present them here in slightly different order for tension headaches.

1. BUTALBITAL COMPOUNDS (FIORINAL, ESGIC, ESGIC PLUS, FIORICET, PHRENILIN)

These are effective but habit-forming medications that should be used no more than once or twice a day. Sedation or euphoria are common.

2. NARCOTICS
CODEINE, HYDROCODONE (VICODIN), PROPOXYPHENE (DARVON, DARVOCET)

These are last-resort medications that are generally not to be used daily and should have strict monthly limits. Your doctor will recommend them only if the milder abortives and daily preventive medications have not worked and your quality of life is significantly compromised by your tension headaches.

3. SEDATIVES
BENZODIAZEPINES, SUCH AS DIAZEPAM (VALIUM) AND CLONAZEPAM (KLONOPIN), AND CHLORDIAZEPOXIDE (LIBRIUM)

These are habit-forming medications that commonly cause sedation. Your doctor should give you a monthly limit and monitor your use; if you need more than the limit, your doctor should switch your medication.

If these medications fail or you take them too often, and you still suffer from severe and frequent daily headaches and feel that your quality of life is seriously compromised by these headaches, your doctor will probably discuss taking preventive medication as well as abortive medication. We discuss this strategy in the next chapter.

9

· · · · · · · ·
〜〜〜

PREVENTING
TENSION HEADACHES

IF YOU'VE TRIED relaxation methods, small to moderate doses of the abortive medications, or are using these medications so often that you're running the risk of getting rebound headaches, don't despair. If your quality of life is still significantly impaired by the frequency and severity of your headaches, preventive medication may be the next step. Many people who switch to preventive medications find that they end up taking less medication and less powerful medication for better relief.

When considering preventive medications, keep in mind the guidelines discussed in Chapter 6.

1. Realize that the goal is moderate improvement with minimal side effects.
2. Be willing to change medications.
3. Try to be tolerant of mildly annoying side effects.
4. Be patient. Many medications take several weeks to become fully effective.
5. Be well informed about each drug you try.

CHOOSING PREVENTIVE MEDICATION

As with other headache situations, finding the right drug to prevent your daily chronic headaches isn't as simple as one would like. You and your doctor will have to consider many factors, such as whether you also get migraines and your sleeping patterns and stomach sensitivity. As in other headache cases, chances are you'll need to take a trial-and-error approach, trying several different medications before you find the right balance of good pain relief with minimal side effects. Again, keep in mind that your goal is to improve your pain by at least 50 to 90 percent with as little medicine as possible.

Many of the medications discussed in this chapter are not specifically indicated for headache by the Food and Drug Administration, as explained in Chapter 1. However, they are commonly used and many doctors and patients have found them helpful. As with our other discussions of medications, this information is meant to serve as a guide only, and you should be sure to check the package insert for complete information about side effects and contraindications.

FIRST-LINE MEDICATIONS FOR PREVENTING TENSION HEADACHES

1. ANTIDEPRESSANTS

These medications are the mainstay therapy for preventing daily headaches and may help whether you are depressed or not. Choosing an antidepressant depends on your anxiety level, age, sleeping patterns, and your tendency to become constipated. Although these medications may also help with depression, they are used here because they benefit headaches, most likely through a serotonin mechanism.

To compare these medications, see the table "The Antidepressants: Comparing Side Effects" and the more complete descriptions with typical dosages in Chapter 6. Here's a quick review of their main differences.

- **AMITRIPTYLINE (ELAVIL)**

Effective for migraines and daily headaches, amitriptyline is inexpensive and can relieve insomnia. Unfortunately, a lot of people can't tolerate its side effects.

SIDE EFFECTS: Sedation, dizziness, a dry mouth, weight gain, and constipation.

- **FLUOXETINE (PROZAC), SERTRALINE (ZOLOFT), OR PAROXETINE (PAXIL)**

All of these medications, which are very similar, pose fewer side effects than amitriptyline, but they are not always as effective for headaches and are more expensive. They are good choices for people who suffer from the blues, a chronic, low-level depression, or for those over fifty, who need a medication with milder side effects.

SIDE EFFECTS: Nausea, anxiety, insomnia, and occasional fatigue. Lack of weight gain (usually) and lack of sedation are major advantages. Reduced sexual desire is common.

- **PROTRIPTYLINE (VIVACTIL)**

Protriptyline is often used when migraines are also a problem. It is nonsedating and does not cause weight gain but is not as effective as amitriptyline.

SIDE EFFECTS: A dry mouth, constipation, and dizziness, but milder than with amitriptyline. Nervousness, insomnia, which can be countered by taking it in the morning, and, less often, blurred vision and stomach upset.

- **NORTRIPTYLINE (PAMELOR, AVENTYL)**

Although better tolerated than amitriptyline, nortriptyline is less effective and more expensive. Often nortriptyline is a first-choice headache preventive for children, adolescents, and the elderly because its side effects are milder. Occasionally helpful for migraines, nortriptyline is usually more effective for chronic daily headache.

SIDE EFFECTS: Similar to amitriptyline but less severe, including sedation (which decreases over time), weight gain, a dry mouth, constipation, and dizziness.

- **DOXEPIN (SINEQUAN)**
  Very similar to amitriptyline, doxepin is more effective than nortriptyline but has stronger side effects.
  SIDE EFFECTS: Sedation, a dry mouth, weight gain, and constipation.

- **DESIPRAMINE (NORPRAMIN)**
  Unlike amitriptyline, fluoxetine, protriptyline, and doxepin, desipramine is not generally useful for migraines but often helps chronic daily headaches. It's very well tolerated but generally not as effective as the other antidepressants. It is sometimes a first choice, however, for people over fifty who might be more sensitive to the antidepressants' side effects.
  SIDE EFFECTS: Sleep disturbances if taken at night; other side effects are similar to amitriptyline but much milder.

- **TRIMIPRAMINE (SURMONTIL)**
  This is a good choice when amitriptyline no longer works (but did), if its side effects were too severe, or if you want a sedative effect. It is well tolerated compared to the other antidepressants, but is sedating. Like desipramine, trimipramine is also used much more commonly for preventing daily headaches than for preventing migraines.
  SIDE EFFECTS: Similar to amitriptyline, including constipation, sedation, a dry mouth, and fatigue.

2. NONSTEROIDAL ANTI-INFLAMMATORIES (NSAIDs)

Commonly used to abort a headache, the NSAIDs are not as effective for preventing headaches as the antidepressants but they do not have the antidepressants' side effects of sedation, a dry mouth, fatigue, and constipation. They do, however, often cause gastrointestinal upset (which you should report to your doctor) and potential damage to the liver and kidneys. They also cost more. Nevertheless, if you are under forty and suffer from arthritis, musculoskeletal problems (painful knees, back, shoulder), menstrual migraines, or the sedating effects of the antidepressants, these medications may be useful. If you are older than forty, these medications are less appropriate for daily use.

Each NSAID has slightly different properties, so if one doesn't work or isn't well tolerated, your doctor may suggest trying another. If you are under age forty, it's probably worthwhile to keep searching for the right one rather than opting for a second-line medication. If you use an NSAID every day, your doctor should monitor you periodically with blood tests to be sure the medication is not causing any liver or kidney damage.

The dosing of these medications varies widely since it is important to maintain the minimum effective amount. General guidelines, however, are indicated in the list of drugs which follows. NSAIDs should always be taken with food. The NSAIDs used commonly to prevent chronic daily headache are also used to prevent migraine headaches and are discussed in more detail in Chapter 6.

- **NAPROXEN (ALEVE, NAPROSYN, ANAPROX):** 500 or 550 mg once or twice a day.
- **FENOPROFEN (NALFON):** 600 to 1,800 mg a day.
- **FLURBIPROFEN (ANSAID):** 100 to 300 mg per day.
- **KETOPROFEN (ORUDIS):** 75 to 150 mg per day.

The following NSAIDs are less commonly used for tension headaches but are sometimes helpful

- **IBUPROFEN (MOTRIN, ADVIL):** Available over the counter; 400 to 1,600 mg per day. (See Chapter 2 for a full discussion.)
- **DICLOFENAC SODIUM (VOLTAREN):** Causes less stomach upset and is possibly more effective than ibuprofen, 75 to 150 mg per day.
- **LODINE:** A newer NSAID that shows great promise, 300 to 600 mg a day.
- **RELAFEN:** Also a newer NSAID. Easier on the stomach, it may be taken once or twice a day, 500 to 1,500 mg.

– **ASPIRIN:** Very inexpensive and available over the counter, two to six pills per day, 650 to 1,950 mg, enteric-coated usually recommended. (See Chapter 2 for a full discussion.)

If neither the antidepressants nor the nonsteroidal anti-inflammatories work to prevent your daily headaches or if you cannot tolerate their side effects, your doctor may suggest one of these second-line preventive medications.

SECOND-LINE MEDICATIONS FOR PREVENTING TENSION HEADACHES

1. VALPROATE (DEPAKOTE)
An often effective seizure medication, valproate is becoming increasing popular in headache treatment. However, it commonly causes gastrointestinal upset, fatigue, and weight gain; hair loss (alopecia) may also occur. (See Chapter 6 for a full discussion.)

2. BETA-BLOCKERS
Beta-blockers, which help prevent blood vessel dilation and may influence serotonin, are occasionally useful for tension headaches. They may, however, cause fatigue, depression, cramps, and weight gain and may interfere with your ability to exercise. The beta-blockers propranolol (Inderal) or nadolol (Corgard) are often combined with a tricyclic antidepressant or an anti-inflammatory. (See Chapter 6 for a full discussion.)

3. MUSCLE RELAXANTS
These are well-tolerated medications but usually only mildly effective. Fatigue is common and limits their usefulness, although caffeine may help counter it. Some of these medications are habit-forming, but they may be used if you have an ulcer, unlike many of the other medications. They are sometimes prescribed

with an NSAID to increase pain relief, and with caffeine to counter fatigue.

• CYCLOBENZAPRINE (FLEXERIL)

This muscle relaxant is one of the most effective for relieving tension headaches, but it may cause severe fatigue.

TYPICAL DOSE: Starting with 5 mg taken at night, increasing up to 10 mg three or four times a day if well tolerated.

SIDE EFFECTS: Drowsiness, dizziness, lightheadedness. Less common are confusion, a dry mouth, rapid heartbeat, and low blood pressure.

• ORPHENADRINE (NORFLEX)

Sometimes effective, this medication is also nonaddicting.

TYPICAL DOSE: 100 mg once or twice a day.

SIDE EFFECTS: Sedation, lightheadedness.

• METHOCARBAMOL (ROBAXIN)

The generic version of this medication is inexpensive, effective, and well tolerated.

TYPICAL DOSE: Starting with 250 mg at night, the dose is slowly increased to 500 or 750 mg one to four times a day.

SIDE EFFECTS: Fatigue, lightheadedness, and dizziness.

4. CALCIUM BLOCKERS (VERAPAMIL)

These medications help prevent blood vessel constriction, which may occur early in a headache, and also influence serotonin. They are occasionally effective but often cause constipation and allergic reactions. Verapamil (Calan, Isoptin, Verelan) is the most effective calcium blocker. (See Chapter 6 for a full discussion.)

If the first- and second-line therapies don't help, there are a few more possible avenues to take.

THIRD-LINE MEDICATIONS FOR PREVENTING TENSION HEADACHES

1. TAKING TWO PREVENTIVE MEDICATIONS

If you are extremely frustrated with moderate or severe headaches and want quick results, or if you suddenly get severe headaches (usually a combination of daily tension headaches and migraines) that you can't deal with, your doctor may suggest pushing the preventive strategy ahead at a faster pace by suggesting that you try two preventive medications. Sometimes when one preventive medication doesn't work, two will. The various preventive medications possess different mechanisms of action.

Common combinations include a tricyclic antidepressant with an NSAID or a beta-blocker; an NSAID with a beta-blocker or a calcium blocker; amitriptyline with propranolol; sometimes valproate (Depakote) with an antidepressant, beta-blocker, or calcium blocker. One or two preventive medications may also be prescribed at the same time as repetitive IV DHE (description follows).

Although the risk of side effects increases with two medications, this treatment is justified if your headaches severely compromise your quality of life.

2. MAO INHIBITORS (PHENELZINE)

Phenelzine (Nardil) is a powerful medication for migraines and daily headaches (and for depression and anxiety). Sometimes it is the only thing that works. Its use is limited, however, because of strict dietary restrictions (see "Third-Line Medications for Preventing Migraines" in Chapter 6.) Some people also object to the common side effects of weight gain and insomnia. Phenelzine is sometimes prescribed with an antidepressant, beta-blocker, calcium blocker, or an NSAID to enhance its efficacy.

3. REPETITIVE IV DHE
Although IV DHE is most effective for migraines, it is some-times useful for daily headaches as well. If you are dependent on analgesics, your doctor may prescribe DHE to help you withdraw from them. It's a safe medication but expensive. (See Chapter 6 for a full discussion.)

4. TRANQUILIZERS
Although only occasionally effective for daily headaches, a tranquilizer is just the right medication for some people. These drugs can, however, be habit-forming so doctors will usually minimize doses and carefully monitor you if you go on one of them.
- **CLONAZEPAM (KLONOPIN)**
  Useful for insomnia and migraines.
- **CHLORDIAZEPOXIDE (LIBRIUM)**
  Relatively mild and well tolerated.
- **DIAZEPAM (VALIUM)**
  Can be useful but habit-forming.
- **PHENOBARBITAL**
  May help with anxiety as well as preventing headaches.

5. AMPHETAMINES
These are last-resort medications that are somewhat effective and generally well tolerated, but they can lead to chemical de-pendency. Insomnia and anxiety are also be potential problems. Typical amphetamines used for preventing tension headaches are methylphenidate (Ritalin), dextroamphetamine (Dexe-drine), or methamphetamine (Desoxyn).

6. DAILY LONG-ACTING NARCOTIC OPIOIDS
The longer-acting opioids, such as methadone (Dolophine), have been used for chronic cancer pain. Methadone, for exam-ple, stays in the bloodstream and remains effective for a longer

period of time than codeine or hydrocodone. It is now being used in some patients with chronic back, neck, or head pain as well. In one recent study conducted at the Robbins Headache Clinic, of forty-four patients with severe daily headaches who had not responded to any previous therapies, two or three tablets of methadone per day significantly helped nineteen patients.

Methadone is generally well tolerated and when used strictly for pain and is unlikely to cause addiction. People do not become euphoric from it, and very few pain patients engage in "drug-seeking" behavior.

TYPICAL DOSE: 5-mg tablet, twice a day.

SIDE EFFECTS: Nausea, fatigue, "spaciness," and constipation; these side effects may limit the use of methadone.

CASE STUDIES

Here are several case studies, showing how all this information on tension headaches might be applied.

PHYLLIS

INITIAL VISIT: Phyllis is a twenty-seven-year-old woman who is home with a young child. She reports that she first began getting chronic daily headaches at sixteen, but they stopped for a few years, from age twenty-two through twenty-four. They have since returned and are now severe. Occasionally Phyllis gets a migraine, but her primary problem is the daily headache. It hurts all over her head as "an aching pressure" and is present all the time, "twenty-four hours a day." She says that over-the-counter medications are of no use. Relaxation techniques do help, but she does not want to do the deep breathing and imaging. The headaches are not increased by any triggers that Phyllis can identify. She says, "Whether I am under no stress or great stress, the headache is there all the time, day after day, and is just the same. It hurts a lot." Chiropractic and massage therapy helped for one or two days, but only minimally. Allergy testing, dental (TMJ) testing, and eye tests were all normal.

Phyllis's doctor prescribes 10 mg of amitriptyline (Elavil) as a preventive medication to be taken at night.

WEEK 6: Phyllis cannot tolerate Elavil because she gained weight and was very tired, even on this low dose. Her doctor prescribes fluoxetine (Prozac), 20 mg each morning, as Prozac usually causes very little sedation or dryness in the mouth.

WEEK 10: Phyllis suffers no side effects from the Prozac, but the medication works only moderately well; she says the pain is "fifty percent" better and wants more relief. Her dose of Prozac is raised to 40 mg a day.

WEEK 13: Phyllis calls her doctor to say she's still getting a headache every day and that the 40 mg of Prozac is making her feel tired and "spacy." The doctor lowers the dose again to 20 mg and prescribes the anti-inflammatory naproxen (anti-inflammatories as preventive medications are prescribed much more in Phyllis's relatively young age range than for older patients).

WEEK 16: Phyllis reports that she is getting no additional relief and the doctor takes her off the naproxen, which carries the risk of gastrointestinal, kidney, and liver side effects. He adds nortriptyline (Pamelor), 10 mg, at night. Phyllis gains some weight, but the headaches are 75 percent improved, and she wishes to stay on Prozac plus Pamelor.

THE FUTURE: If Phyllis is willing, she can try other preventive medications, such as other antidepressants or valproate (Depakote), but she prefers to stick with her current regimen for now. Beta-blockers, such as propranolol, are also possibilities.

HEATHER

INITIAL VISIT: Heather is a thirty-three-year-old stockbroker with a history of severe daily tension headache and one migraine monthly. She's had the daily headaches since age sixteen, but they didn't become severe until two years ago. Her job is very stressful, as is her marriage. When Heather saw a physician last year, she was taking sixteen aspirin plus over-the-counter caffeine tablets and six ibuprofen tablets a day. Her blood tests revealed that her liver was irritated and she was having severe stomach pains due to the stress and medicine.

Heather's physician took her off the aspirin and ibuprofen and prescribed Esgic (a butalbital compound with acetaminophen and caffeine), but Heather is now consuming ten Esgic tablets a day.

She is experiencing some degree of analgesic rebound headache, in which her medication is actually creating more pain for her the next day. This is a common problem and usually occurs when someone takes more than four or five pain relievers (though can range from as little as two to as many as eight) a day.

Heather tapers off the painkillers and gets four injections of intravenous DHE, which is commonly used to help people withdraw from analgesics and to relieve the headaches for a period of time. The key with Heather is to avoid painkillers and to find an effective daily preventive medication.

The physician prescribes nortriptyline (Pamelor), a tricyclic antidepressant that is somewhat milder than amitriptyline (Elavil). They hope that the medication will prevent both the daily tension headache as well as the monthly migraine. Heather also receives a prescription for ergotamine (Cafergot) for the migraines, but the plan is simply to use preventive medications for her daily pain.

WEEK 4: Heather has successfully withdrawn from the analgesics with the DHE breaking the cycle of rebound headaches. The nortriptyline has helped prevent headaches, but her blood tests continue to show some liver irritation, which may have been caused by the nortriptyline. Her daily preventive medication is changed to fluoxetine (Prozac), one capsule each morning.

WEEK 6: The Prozac is not helping, so the dose is raised to two capsules each morning. The liver tests have returned to normal. Heather is not allowed to consume any daily painkillers.

WEEK 7: The tension headaches are only about 25 percent improved with the Prozac, so Heather switches back to nortriptyline and the dose is slowly increased to the point at which the headaches are 70 percent improved in severity. Her liver tests remain normal. The monthly migraines are gone.

Analgesic rebound headaches can be relatively easily controlled once someone is no longer taking pain medications. The keys are to find a preventive medication that will work. In rare situations, in which all of the prevention approaches have failed, daily pain medications may be used in controlled amounts; twelve or fourteen tablets of an analgesic per day is unacceptable. Heather receives DHE in the nasal spray form to take for an occasional migraine if Cafergot does not help.

THE FUTURE: If the nortriptyline stops working or produces unacceptable side effects in the future, there are many other options, including other antidepressants; beta-blockers, such as propranolol (Inderal); verapamil (Isoptin); and valproate (Depakote). If none of these approaches are successful, either alone or in combination, stronger medications, such as MAO inhibitors (Nardil) or even a stimulant (Ritalin), may help. However, these are considered end-of-the-line treatments. For her migraines, Heather may consider Imitrex injections.

LOUIS

INITIAL VISIT: Louis, a forty-two-year-old accountant, has had daily headaches for almost two decades. They hurt in a "hatband" fashion around his head and increase in severity as the day goes on. He reports that they are worse with stress and weather changes, if he drinks red wine, or if he eats food that contains MSG. The headaches wax and wane, and occasionally Louis goes four or five days without one.

For four years, Louis used two Excedrin Extra-Strength tablets a day to control his pain. Relaxation techniques and exercise have not helped. Massage helps for one day, but then the pain returns. Louis has sought relief, but to no avail, from chiropractors, allergists, dentists, sinus doctors, and eye doctors.

He began needing more and more Excedrin, to the point of taking eight a day. His stomach began to hurt (due to the aspirin in the Excedrin) and his headaches were getting worse. All the Excedrin was evidently giving Louis rebound headaches. His doctor takes him off Excedrin and places him on an antidepressant as preventive medication, protriptyline (Vivactil). The doctor chooses Vivactil over amitriptyline because it is not sedating and never causes weight gain; he chooses it over fluoxetine (Prozac) because it is more effective. Vivactil can keep people up at night, but Louis does not have a problem with insomnia.

TWO MONTHS LATER: On Vivactil, the headaches decrease to the point where Louis has almost no pain, but he has side effects from the medication, particularly constipation, a dry mouth, and insomnia. His doctor prescribes the beta-blocker, propranolol (Inderal), instead. While Prozac is still a possibility, Louis and his doctor decide not to continue with an antidepressant for now because of Louis's problems with Vivactil's side effects.

THREE MONTHS LATER: Although Louis hasn't called the office between visits, he now reports that the Inderal helped only a bit. On his own, he went back to taking aspirin and caffeine in the form of Anacin. Once again he crept up to taking eight a day, and once more the headaches increased because of the analgesic rebound situation. A stressful divorce further increased the headaches, and Louis began mixing ibuprofen with the aspirin and caffeine. He developed an ulcer and was hospitalized. At this point, his doctor takes him off the analgesics and gives him five injections of IV DHE, which greatly helps the headaches. The doctor prescribes nortriptyline (Pamelor), a mild antidepressant, 25 mg at night, as a preventive medication. This dose is low. As nortriptyline may cause constipation (and a dry mouth), Louis's doctor informs him about how to minimize this problem through a proper diet and laxatives if necessary.

TWO MONTHS LATER: Louis reports that he does get a mild dry mouth from the medication, but that the preventive medication (the antidepressant with no analgesics) is quite successful in that he is now getting relatively few headaches. He estimates that the pain is 80 percent better. Because this improvement is within the range of success expected with preventive medications, Louis agrees to continue on the nortriptyline. Although weight gain with nortriptyline can be a major problem, it is not in Louis's case.

THE FUTURE: If the current dose of nortriptyline begins to lose its effectiveness, the doctor may increase the dose. Or he and Louis may want to consider valproate (Depakote). Alternative antidepressants, such as Prozac or Zoloft, may also help.

JOSEPH

INITIAL VISIT: Joseph is a sixty-eight-year-old executive with a history of chronic daily headache, moderate in intensity, and frequent, sharp pains in the back of his head, on the right side only, lasting up to one minute. The sharp pains are diagnosed as occipital neuralgia (to read more about this condition, see Chapter 12). Joseph has had headaches since he was twenty-six, but they have gotten worse in the past several years. Stress, certain foods, and golf exacerbate them. His mother and two of his three children have a history of headaches. Joseph has had ulcers and has high blood pressure. He reports that over-the-counter medications have ceased working for him and that he has tried several prescription acetaminophen-based analgesics, but none of them has been effective.

Joseph's doctor instructs him in the nonmedication aspects of headaches, but relaxation techniques are generally ineffective for his age range. The doctor prescribes propranolol (Inderal), a high blood pressure medication, as a preventive. Because of Joseph's advanced age, the doctor keeps the dose low to minimize side effects. Although an antidepressant may be more effective, Joseph's doctor chooses propranolol to lessen his medication over the long term and because it should stabilize his blood pressure as well.

For an abortive medication, Joseph receives a prescription for butalbital with acetaminophen (Phrenilin) and instructions to take no more than two per day. Any more could lead to rebound headaches. To alleviate the sharp pains in the back of his head, Joseph gets an injection of novocaine (Marcaine) in that area. This procedure is easy and safe and takes just minutes in the doctor's office yet it can provide weeks or even months of relief.

WEEK 4: Joseph reports that his headaches are about 20 percent better on the Inderal. His blood pressure is under control. The novocaine injection provided three weeks of relief for the pains in the back of the head, but they have started to return. The doctor increases the Inderal dose.

WEEK 6: Joseph calls to say the increased dose does not help and leaves him tired. The doctor reduces the Inderal dose. To supplement Joseph's preventive medication, the doctor prescribes nortriptyline (10 mg of Pamelor, quickly raised to 25 mg), a mild antidepressant, to take at night because it helps sleeping. The Phrenilin is continued as an abortive, to be taken when needed.

WEEK 12: Joseph calls to say his headaches are 70 percent better, but he is very tired and constipated. These side effects are from the Pamelor, so the doctor lowers the dose back to 10 mg.

Joseph also reports that the Phrenilin no longer relieves the headache once it starts, so he and his doctor agree that he should discontinue the medication and stick to daily preventives. Because of his ulcer problems, Joseph can't use aspirin or anti-inflammatories as abortives, and many of the other choices are too strong and cause too many side effects. The aspirin-NSAID medications are prescribed infrequently for older people because of the increased risk of side effects with advancing age. Joseph and his doctor discuss the possibility of a very small amount of daily narcotic analgesic, such as hydrocodone, but they consider it a last resort. For now, Joseph will use the daily preventives and not chase after the pain every four hours.

WEEK 16: Joseph reports that his headaches are about 40 percent better than they were before his first visit. The low 10-mg dose of Pamelor helps somewhat and does not make him tired. He remains on the Inderal for the blood pressure and headaches.

THE FUTURE: Other considerations, if needed, may be one of the newer antidepressants, such as Prozac, Zoloft, or Paxil, all of which are used for headaches. These medications have been very useful because they generally do not cause sedation, weight gain, or constipation. However, they do have some side effects, such as anxiety, nausea, decreased libido or sexual performance, and insomnia. In addition, other blood pressure medications may help Joseph, such as different beta-blockers (Corgard, Lopressor, Tenormin) or calcium blockers (Isoptin, Calan).

10
. . . .

UNDERSTANDING
AND TREATING
CLUSTER HEADACHES

CLUSTER HEADACHES, though rare, are one of the most painful experiences known to humankind. If you are one of the unfortunate few who gets them, you may suffer terribly, as they can be excruciating and debilitating. The pain may last anywhere from fifteen minutes to three hours, occasionally longer. Usually, the pain sears through or around one eye, or locates itself in the temple. These headaches are called cluster headaches because they occur in waves, a series of headaches lasting several weeks to several months, once or twice a year, most commonly in the spring and fall. Occasionally, the intervals between attacks are much longer.

WHAT ARE CLUSTER HEADACHES?

Six times more common among men than women, cluster headaches cause extreme and sudden pain without any warning or aura. Although experts assume that serotonin imbalances cause clusters, they also think that a malfunctioning of the body's biological clock, the hypothalamus, may also be involved because of the cyclic nature of these headaches. Cluster headaches are probably one of the vascular headaches, as are migraines, partly caused by constricting and dilating blood vessels — probably of the carotid artery close to the eye — but surrounding nerves are also involved. Since smokers have a higher rate of cluster headaches, subtle changes in the bloodstream that may occur in smokers probably also play a role.

Usually cluster headaches start between ages twenty and forty-five. If you first got cluster headaches early in life, chances are you will outgrow them by your forties; people who start getting cluster headaches later in life have a greater chance of having chronic cluster headaches.

A cluster headache often begins with a sense of fullness in one ear and then progresses to a stab of pain near the eye, forehead, or cheek, sometimes even as low as the jaw. Within minutes, the pain can become excruciating. For most people, the pain remains on the same side, though occasionally it may switch to the other, either during the same cluster cycle or in the next cycle. Your eye will probably tear and your nose will run on the same side as the pain.

On average, attacks last forty-five minutes, starting at the same time of day, usually during the night. Typically, they build in intensity over days or weeks. The series of headaches most commonly consists of one or two headaches a day for three to eight weeks (sometimes for as long as five months), once or twice a year. These clusters are called "intermittent" or "episodic." About one in ten sufferers has "chronic" cluster headaches, with less than a six-month break between cycles.

The pain may be extremely intense, "like an eye is being pulled out." Many people writhe in agony, rock, or bang their heads against the wall. Some sufferers say that the pain is worse than it would be if a limb were cut off in an accident.

Cluster headaches are often misdiagnosed as a sinus or allergy problem because of the runny or stuffed nose and teary eye. You can probably identify your headaches as clusters if they follow this pattern:

- Onset between ages twenty and forty-five
- Most common among men (six times more than women)
- Occur same time of year, with no headache between the cluster cycles
- Attacks usually occur at night
- During a cycle, alcohol is the most common trigger
- Severe, excruciating pain on one side, usually around the eye
- Eye tearing (lacrimation) and red on the side of the pain
- Small pupil (miosis of the pupil)
- Drooping eyelid
- Stuffed or runny nostril on the side of the pain
- Sweaty face or forehead

NONDRUG STRATEGIES TO TREAT CLUSTER HEADACHES

Unfortunately, very little except medication really helps cluster headaches. The pain is too severe for relaxation methods, although a few simple deep-breathing exercises can help you cope with the dread and anticipation of another cluster. People in the midst of a series are often extremely anxious, fearing a night of intense, excruciating pain.

Applying ice to the painful area may help, although some people prefer heat. A hot shower massager with moderate pressure on the scalp may also ease some pain.

Once a cluster series has started, sensitivity to alcohol is much greater and often can trigger an attack. The other typical headache foods are less important, although you should avoid especially MSG, and to some extent, aged cheeses, aged meats, and chocolate during a cluster series. Occasionally, certain triggers, such as the letdown after stress, excessive cold or heat, or bright light may bring on a cluster. By and large, however, you can't control the time when a cluster will strike, except perhaps with medication.

TREATING CLUSTERS WITH MEDICATION

If you get either intermittent or chronic cluster headaches, you will probably cope best if you have medication both to treat and to prevent an attack. Since the pain is very sudden, intense, and relatively brief, lasting less than an hour, the abortive medication must act quickly. Taking medication by mouth usually isn't fast enough. An oral pain reliever is more useful if your attacks typically last more than an hour. Antinausea medication is sometimes used, not only to combat nausea but for its sedative effect as well.

FIRST-LINE MEDICATIONS FOR
ABORTING CLUSTER HEADACHES

When you first go to a doctor about cluster headaches, chances are that he will recommend one of these treatments to relieve the pain after the headache has started.

1. OXYGEN
This treatment involves inhaling oxygen from a tank. It is very effective in 80 percent of cases and renting a tank and mask is relatively easy and moderately inexpensive.

To use the oxygen tank, sit, leaning slightly forward. Inhale 100 percent oxygen (8 liters per minute) with the mask, for fifteen to twenty minutes, longer if needed, but no more than one hour a day, assuming you have no pulmonary problems.

2. ERGOTAMINE TARTRATE
A moderately effective blood vessel constrictor, ergotamine tartrate has many side effects, especially severe anxiety and nausea. Although this medication presents the risk of rebound

headaches when used with migraines, they do not occur with cluster headaches.

Unlike sumatriptan and DHE, in which the most effective form is an injection, ergotamine tartrate can be effective in pill form, though suppositories are most effective. After age forty, this medication must be used with caution because of the risk for heart complications.

For details about specific medications in this group (Cafergot pills and suppositories), see "Second-Line Medications for Aborting Migraines" in Chapter 5.

3. SUMATRIPTAN (IMITREX)

Sumatriptan, a relatively new medication, is extremely effective when it is injected, but the premeasured, convenient auto-injectors are expensive. In pill form, sumatriptan is much less expensive but also less effective.

If you are willing to press the auto-injector against your arm or leg and push a button to release a small needle, then sumatriptan will be particularly useful for you because it is so effective and appears to be very safe. It does cause nausea, however, in some people. Its risks increase with age, and if you are over forty-five, your doctor will check you for heart risk factors. If you are over sixty-five, chances are your doctor will not recommend this medication. Sumatriptan is also not recommended for pregnant or nursing women, children, adolescents, and people with liver, kidney, or cardiovascular problems. This medication is often prescribed in combination with oxygen and a pain reliever.

The long-term safety of daily use is not yet known. Therefore, no more than six injections a week are now recommended. People who need sumatriptan daily for more than one or two months, should explore other options.

SIDE EFFECTS: Relatively mild (milder than with DHE) pain around the injection site (using ice beforehand can help), temporary sensation changes, such as taste disturbances, nausea, tingling, hot flashes, feelings of pressure anywhere on body, chest discomfort (believed to be unrelated to the heart), dizziness, and overall weakness and drowsiness.

See Chapter 5 for more details.

4. DIHYDROERGOTAMINE (DHE)

Similar to sumatriptan, DHE is somewhat less effective but lasts longer and has been on the market for years. (DHE is more effective than ergotamine.) Unlike sumatriptan, it is not available in premeasured auto-injectors or in pill form, though it is available in a nasal spray. Injections, however, are the most effective form.

If you have any kind of heart disease, DHE must be used with caution. For more details, see "Second-Line Medications for Aborting Migraines" in Chapter 5.

SECOND-LINE MEDICATIONS FOR
ABORTING CLUSTER HEADACHES

When the first-line medications don't work, there are other options.

1. PAIN RELIEVERS

At this stage of headache management, the doctor may suggest anything ranging from over-the-counter Excedrin Extra-Strength to naproxen (Anaprox DS), Norgesic Forte, butalbital compounds (Fiorinal or Esgic), or perhaps narcotics, all of which we discuss in detail in Chapter 5. Because addiction is always a potential problem with narcotics, you should resort to them only when the milder options don't work.

2. LIDOCAINE NASAL SPRAY

Though rarely useful by itself for treating clusters, Lidocaine spray may be recommended in combination with other methods. It is mildly effective but safe, easy to use, and has minimal side effects.

TYPICAL DOSE: The pharmacist will put 4 percent Lidocaine (from a bottle) into a plastic nasal spray container. Lie down, with your head extended back, and turn your head toward the side of the pain. Spray two or three times but no more than eight in twenty-four hours. If a spray bottle is unavailable, 1 ml of 4 percent Lidocaine can be dropped with an eye dropper into the nostril near the pain.

SIDE EFFECTS: Sometimes temporary numbness in the throat. Nervousness and rapid heartbeat occur rarely.

3. KETOROLAC (TORADOL) INJECTIONS

Ketorolac is relatively expensive (about $10 an injection), but it is an effective and fast-acting anti-inflammatory when injected. It is nonsedating and nonaddictive and is available in pill form but but must be injected for most effective relief. Prefilled syringes are available.

TYPICAL DOSE: 60 mg in a prefilled syringe, repeated half an hour or an hour later if needed, with 30 mg or 60 mg. No more than three injections per week.

SIDE EFFECTS: Use should be monitored and limited during a series of cluster headaches, to avoid kidney and liver complications. Because ketorolac is an anti-inflammatory, it may cause stomach pain.

See Chapter 5 for more details.

4. ANTINAUSEA MEDICATION

These medications can help any nausea that occurs, as well as promote sedation, which is sometimes desired to tolerate the cluster.

- **PROMETHAZINE (PHENERGAN)**
  Promethazine is sedating but has few other side effects. Available in pill or suppository form, promethazine also helps enhance the effectiveness of pain relievers.
- **PROCHLORPERAZINE (COMPAZINE) AND CHLORPROMAZINE (THORAZINE)**
  These are stronger antinausea medications that are useful to promote sedation when you want to avoid going to the emergency room for your pain.
  See Chapter 5 for more details.

PREVENTING CLUSTER HEADACHES

When abortive medications don't relieve your cluster headaches and your headaches occur daily for longer than fifteen minutes, most doctors will recommend a preventive. You may choose to take daily preventive medication as soon as a series begins because the headaches are extremely severe and difficult to relieve when in progress. But to take preventive medications, you must be willing to take daily medicine for the length of the cluster series and endure the possible side effects. If you get chronic, rather than intermittent, cluster headaches, you'll probably do best if you take daily medication year-round.

Once you are certain that a cluster cycle has begun, your doctor may recommend that you start taking cortisone, the fastest-acting of the first-line preventive medications, along with another medication in this group, either lithium or verapamil. The theory is that by the time the cortisone is withdrawn (it shouldn't be taken for too long), the second preventive will have become effective.

When your cluster series ends, the medication can be stopped a week or two after the last headache and not started up again until the first signs of another series. After discovering what's effective and tolerable for you, your doctor will probably recommend that you institute the same regimen whenever you think a cluster series is beginning.

FIRST-LINE MEDICATIONS FOR PREVENTING CLUSTER HEADACHES

As with migraines, the effects of these medications are cumulative, so if one medication is not completely effective, the doctor may recommend a combination of verapamil, lithium, and cortisone. Lithium with verapamil is a common combination for clusters, with or without using cortisone for brief periods.

1. CORTISONE
Prednisone, dexamethasone (Decadron), triamcinolone (Aristocort), or an injectable form (ACTH gel or Depo-Medrol)

Cortisone is very effective and used primarily for episodic clusters. Side effects are likely, as your physician and medication package insert will explain. Cluster headache sufferers usually take cortisone for just one or two weeks during the peak of the series.

TYPICAL DOSE: Should be as small as possible and taken with food. Prednisone, 20 mg (or Decadron, 4 mg) once a day for three days, then 10 mg of Prednisone (half a pill) per day for six to ten days. Injectable forms provide quick relief for up to a week, usually not longer. Additional cortisone may be used later in the cycle if the clusters increase.

SIDE EFFECTS: Nervousness, moodiness, and sleep problems; when used for brief periods, side effects are usually minimal. Sometimes fluid retention, fatigue, gastrointestinal upset, and stomach pain.

2. VERAPAMIL (CALAN, ISOPTIN, VERELAN)
Verapamil is a well-tolerated calcium blocker with minimal side effects, though it may aggravate or cause chronic daily headaches. It is effective for episodic and chronic clusters, but

needs to be taken for at least several days and sometimes several weeks to become fully effective.

TYPICAL DOSE: 240 mg slow-release or long-acting pill once or twice a day. At the start of a headache, verapamil is often prescribed with cortisone and then still taken after cortisone is discontinued.

SIDE EFFECTS: Constipation, allergic reactions (rashes), dizziness, insomnia, anxiety, and occasionally fatigue.

3. LITHIUM

Lithium is well tolerated when taken in low doses. It can be very helpful for chronic clusters and, to a lesser degree, episodic clusters. It is commonly combined with verapamil or cortisone.

TYPICAL DOSE: 300 to 900 mg a day, occasionally higher.

SIDE EFFECTS: Drowsiness, mood swings, nausea, vomiting, thirst, tremor, diarrhea. Low doses and good monitoring usually avoid serious problems than can occur otherwise.

SECOND-LINE MEDICATIONS FOR PREVENTING CLUSTER HEADACHES

When first-line medications do not reliably prevent cluster headaches, a physician may progress to one of these medications, which we describe in more detail earlier in the book.

1. METHYSERGIDE (SANSERT)

Somewhat effective for episodic clusters but not usually for chronic clusters, Sansert can be useful but has many potential side effects, such as nausea, leg cramps, and dizziness. It is not, however, generally recommended for people with active peptic ulcers, peripheral vascular disease, cardiac valve problems, coronary artery disease, high blood pressure, kidney or liver problems, or for those who are pregnant or over forty-five. See Chapter 6 for a full discussion.

2. VALPROATE (DEPAKOTE)

A seizure medication that is often used for cluster, migraine, and tension headaches, valproate is sometimes very useful but it may cause lethargy, gastrointestinal upset, mood swings, weight gain, and hair loss.

It is fairly well tolerated, but nausea, gastritis (stomach pain or burning), sedation, emotional upset (depression or mood swings), hair loss, rashes, and dose-related tremors are relatively common. If taken for months, weight gain is common. Liver functions and blood counts need to be monitored closely in the first several months, but for episodic clusters the entire duration of use is only one or two months, and one blood test is usually adequate. See Chapter 6 for a full discussion.

3. ERGOTAMINES (CAFERGOT, BELLERGAL-S)

While headache doctors do not usually prescribe daily ergotamines, blood vessel constrictors, because of the risk of long-term effects and rebound headaches (common in migraine patients), the risk is much smaller in cluster sufferers who typically use the medication for a briefer period, only four to eight weeks, and stop after an episode is over.

Great caution must be taken by people who are older than age forty or forty-five. Ergotamines are not usually recommended for anyone with high blood pressure, heart disease, or vascular disease in the legs.

TYPICAL DOSE: Most effective when taken within several hours of the expected cluster attack. If a headache typically occurs at eleven P.M., then optimal timing of the drug is nine or ten P.M. The usual dose is 1 or 2 mg (up to 4 mg) per day.

- **CAFERGOT** pills or suppositories may be used as the source of ergotamine, but the 100 mg of caffeine increases side effects.
- **BELLERGAL-S** is comprised of ergotamine, phenobarbital (a sedative), and belladonna. The sedating effect of phenobarbital is occasionally helpful for the cluster patient, but the rela-

tively low dose of ergotamine (0.6 mg) is usually insufficient to prevent an attack.

SIDE EFFECTS: Nausea and nervousness, fatigue, muscle aches, tingling, numbing in the hands or feet, chest pain. See Chapter 5 for more details.

4. ERGONOVINE (ERGOTRATE)

A well-tolerated medication, ergonovine is generally not as effective as methysergide but it poses fewer side effects.

TYPICAL DOSE: 0.2 mg, two to four times a day.

SIDE EFFECTS: Mild gastrointestinal upset, anxiety.

5. STEROID BLOCKADE OF THE OCCIPITAL NERVE (CORTISONE)

When other drugs cannot control a headache, sufferers can use this therapy at the peak of the series. By placing cortisone (such as Depo-Medrol or betamethasone) in the region of the greater occipital nerve, a cluster can be relieved somewhat for up to weeks at a time. These medications are well tolerated, with few side effects.

TYPICAL DOSE: 60 to 80 mg of Depo-Medrol per injection. An injection may be repeated once, if necessary, but two injections per cluster series is generally the maximum.

SIDE EFFECTS: Infection, discoloration or dimpling of skin, though rare, may occur.

For a full discussion on treating occipital neuralgia, see Chapter 12.

THIRD-LINE MEDICATIONS FOR
PREVENTING EPISODIC CLUSTER HEADACHES

If none of these strategies works for you, your doctor may recommend either intravenous DHE, administered repetitively, or a cocaine solution to be used nasally during the day to prevent the clusters.

1. INTRAVENOUS DIHYDROERGOTAMINE (IV DHE)

IV DHE can quickly cut down on the number of cluster headaches you get and can control clusters while you wait for a preventive medication (such as verapamil or lithium) to take effect. Its pain-relieving effects may last for weeks.

See Chapter 6 for a full discussion of IV DHE.

2. COCAINE SOLUTION

If your episodic cluster series lasts several months and all other preventive measures have failed, cocaine may help you. It is particularly useful during a peak season of chronic clusters. The treatment involves using a 10 percent solution during the day to reduce the number and severity of the clusters. This dose rarely produces any euphoric or cognitive effects.

Addiction risk may be a problem (and its use generally would not be recommended if you have any addiction history), but the low concentration, high cost, and difficulty in obtaining the solution makes cocaine a last-resort therapy.

TYPICAL DOSE: One or two drops in each nostril one to four times a day. If the clusters are severe and out of control, your doctor may suggest beginning with two drops four times a day, quickly cutting the dose down to as little as is effective. Usually limited to two grams of cocaine in two months.

SIDE EFFECTS: Occasional nervousness or insomnia; euphoric effects of cocaine may occur but not commonly. If euphoria is experienced, the percentage of cocaine should be cut down to 4 percent or stopped completely. The patient must understand the addiction potential.

ADDITIONAL TREATMENTS FOR
EPISODIC CLUSTER HEADACHES

Occasionally, other medications may help cluster headaches, including indomethacin, phenelzine, cyproheptadine, nifedipine, and beta-blockers, such as propranolol.

• **Indomethacin (Indocin)**, an anti-inflammatory, occasionally reduces the number of cluster headaches. See Chapter 12 on "Chronic Paroxysmal Hemicrania," a rare form of clusters in which the headaches are infrequent but very brief.

• **Phenelzine (Nardil)**, an MAO inhibitor, is a powerful anti-migraine medication that is occasionally useful for cluster headaches. See Chapter 6 for more details.

• **Cyproheptadine (Periactin)** is occasionally helpful for clusters, but its effect is usually very mild. Side effects, such as fatigue and weight gain, are often problems. Best when used with other therapies for clusters.

• **Nifedipine (Procardia)**, a well-tolerated calcium blocker, is as effective as verapamil for many cluster patients. However, if verapamil does not work, the nifedipine usually is ineffective as well. The usual dose is 60 mg per day divided into two to three doses. Its side effects are very similar to those of verapamil.

• **Beta-blockers** are, at times, mildly effective for cluster patients, but much less effective generally than the usual cluster therapies. Propranolol (Inderal) or nadolol (Corgard) are discussed in Chapter 6.

ADDITIONAL TREATMENTS FOR
PREVENTING CHRONIC CLUSTER HEADACHES

To prevent chronic cluster headaches, a doctor will probably use the same treatments as for episodic clusters. When nothing else seems effective and the pain is consistently on the same side, then the doctor may suggest a surgical technique conducted at only a few medical centers.

Radiofrequency trigeminal rhizotomy kills trigeminal nerve fibers involved in pain conduction, but sometimes the procedure must be repeated to be effective. A specialized technique, the surgery is conducted primarily at the Houston Headache Clinic under the supervision of Dr. Ninan Mathew. **Retrogasserian injection of glycerol** is a new and promising technique as well.

CASE STUDIES

As we have discussed, medication for clusters is used only during the cluster cycle and not in between. Abortive medication offers some relief once the clusters begin, and preventive medication helps avoid potentially disabling and excruciating pain. Here are several typical cluster headache cases.

RICHARD

INITIAL VISIT: Richard, a forty-year-old lawyer, has a five-year history of suffering from five weeks of cluster headaches each fall. The cluster period begins slowly, increasing over one week and reaching a peak in which Richard has two or three severe cluster attacks each day. They occur between ten P.M. and three A.M. and last forty to ninety minutes. The pain is always on the right side, with the eye tearing and right nostril congested.

He is now one week into his fall cluster series. The headaches are increasing in intensity, and he is miserable with the pain. Richard's doctor prescribes abortive medication to ease an attack in progress as well as a preventive regimen.

Richard and his doctor discuss using oxygen as an abortive,

but Richard prefers to try Cafergot tablets first. He has no risk factors for ergotamines and is reluctant to self-inject DHE or sumatriptan. He will take one Cafergot at the beginning of the cluster and apply ice to the painful area.

For preventive therapy, the doctor prescribes 20 mg of Prednisone (cortisone or corticosteroid) in the morning and one with dinner, or 40 mg per day for four days, to be reduced gradually over the next two weeks. By tapering this medication quickly, Richard avoids the risk of serious side effects and he can reserve the medication for use later in the cluster period, if necessary. If Richard were taking medium to high cortisone doses for three weeks, it would not be safe to use even more cortisone, so he keeps his use to a minimum.

Along with the cortisone, the doctor prescribes 240 mg of the calcium blocker verapamil, hoping that by the time the Prednisone is tapered and discontinued, the verapamil will have become effective.

DAY 6: Richard reports that he had five very good days, but as the Prednisone is decreased, the headaches become more severe. Cafergot does not help; last night he had ninety minutes of extreme pain. Richard now agrees to give oxygen a try and rents a tank. The doctor gives him a plastic spray bottle of topical Lidocaine, 4 percent, to use as needed on the side of the pain. He is to lie supine, turn his head toward the side of the pain, extend it back, and spray two or three times into the nostril as needed. While Lidocaine is only somewhat effective for cluster headaches, side effects are minimal. Even just 25 percent relief makes the Lidocaine worthwhile.

Richard is to continue decreasing the Prednisone, with a now doubled dose of verapamil (480 mg per day) to maintain the preventive therapy.

DAY 10: Now in the third week of what is expected to be a five-week cycle, Richard reports that the oxygen helps, but Lidocaine does not. The clusters are less severe but continue to occur twice a night. The verapamil may be having some effect. He is down to 20 mg per day of Prednisone, and he and his doctor decide to taper off the Prednisone over the next six days. If the headaches get dramatically worse, he can increase it again. Richard agrees to come into the office two days in a row for IV DHE, which takes three hours per treatment.

DAY 14: Richard had complete relief for four days, and then the headaches returned but were not nearly as severe.

DAY 20: The headaches are gone, and after one week Richard tapers off the verapamil over six days. If the headaches return during those six days, he will increase the verapamil again, to 480 mg per day, and may reinstitute the Prednisone.

THE FUTURE: The next time Richard's cluster period begins, he will use oxygen as an abortive and will strongly consider self-injections of sumatriptan or DHE. He will begin taking verapamil and about two weeks' worth of Prednisone. Richard may again use IV DHE to ease the severity of the clusters during his peak period of headaches.

SHELDON

INITIAL VISIT: Sheldon is a fifty-five-year-old insurance salesman who has been getting episodic cluster headaches once or twice a year ever since he was twenty-six. They usually occur for six or eight weeks, in the spring and fall, with two to four headaches per twenty-four hours. The headaches are always around Sheldon's left eye, with tearing, running of the left nostril, and tenderness in the back of his head. The pain typically begins at ten or eleven P.M. and often awakens him from sleep. The headache lasts two hours and is sharp and extremely debilitating. Sheldon feels completely incapacitated during the headache cycle. His dad had migraines. Sheldon smokes cigarettes. Alcohol and MSG trigger increased headaches during the cluster cycle, but outside of the cycle, Sheldon never experiences a cluster headache.

Cortisone medication (Decadron, Medrol, Prednisone) was effective for a number of years as a preventive used during the cluster period, but it no longer helps. Methysergide (Sansert) did not help, and verapamil (Isoptin, Calan) helped until last year, but is no longer effective.

One week into the cluster series, Sheldon is placed on lithium, 600 mg (two pills), as a preventive medication to be taken at dinnertime because his headaches occur primarily at night. His doctor teaches him how to self-inject sumatriptan (Imitrex), which helps the vast majority of cluster sufferers. Imitrex is expensive, but it often stops the cluster pain within minutes. Sheldon also receives a small tank of oxygen, to breathe eight liters per minute, as needed, by mask. Sheldon is instructed to quit smoking gradually, as this often will cut down on the clusters.

WEEK 3: Sheldon reports that the clusters have decreased with the lithium, down to one every other night. The Imitrex does stop the clusters within ten minutes, but the oxygen helps only a little. Sheldon does not want to use Imitrex for every headache, so the doctor prescribes the butalbital compound Fiorinal as a pain reliever. While the analgesics, such as Fiorinal, are not ideal for treating clusters, they are useful at times. The pain pills do take at least twenty to thirty minutes to become effective.

WEEK 8: Sheldon reports that the lithium was helpful for four weeks but then ceased being effective. The dose is increased to three pills per day.

WEEK 9: The increased dose of lithium still does not help. The doctor prescribes a beta-blocker, propranolol (Inderal), which is occasionally useful for clusters. Because Sheldon is fifty-five, Inderal is safer for him than daily ergotamines or valproate (Depakote). If the Inderal is not effective, however, Sheldon's doctor might consider trying Depakote next.

WEEK 10: The Inderal is not effective. Sheldon decides that because the headache cycle is due to end soon, he will simply use abortive medications — Imitrex injections, oxygen, and Fiorinal — and not pursue preventive measures.

THE FUTURE: When the next cycle begins, Depakote will be a very reasonable preventive alternative for Sheldon. The other medications have either stopped working or never worked for him. He will continue to take Fiorinal and Imitrex as abortives.

11

········

HEADACHES
IN CHILDREN

WITNESSING your child endure the pain of headaches can be particularly difficult. For one thing, it is always hard to see your children in pain. In the case of headaches, you may feel guilty that something you did, such as arguing with them or with a spouse, may have contributed to their distress. Or you may get headaches yourself and worry that your child may develop a similar pattern. You may also feel helpless, not quite sure how you can aid your child in pain.

When your child has frequent headaches, it can be hard on the entire family. He may miss a lot of school, his siblings may complain over the attention he is getting, or the sick child may relish all the extra attention and then exaggerate his head pain to keep getting more. Adolescents who get severe, frequent headaches often become depressed, and that can affect the whole family, too.

Although headaches are difficult illnesses, especially in children, you can rest assured: many nondrug strategies can help prevent headaches in children, and when medication is needed to relieve pain and restore the quality of life, there is a safe and effective arsenal from which to draw.

WHO GETS HEADACHES?

Unfortunately, many children get headaches. Head pain accounts for more than a million lost days of school every year. Even two-year-olds can get migraines, although they often are misdiagnosed as flu symptoms. Age six is a more typical time for migraines to start, especially among boys. By age seven, some 40 percent of children will have had a headache; most are tension (muscle contraction) headaches. By age ten, 4 percent have had a migraine. After age twelve, many boys outgrow childhood migraines, while girls start getting more of them as their hormones change. All told, about one in ten children may suffer from migraines.

SYMPTOMS IN CHILDREN

If your family has a history of migraines and your child gets severe headaches, there is a good chance that he's inherited his headaches and that they're migraines. Other clues leading to migraines are headaches associated with nausea, visual auras, or typical migraine triggers, such as particular foods or stress. The stress that triggers migraines may not always be "bad stress" but may be "good stress," such as the excitement of a birthday party or a special trip.

Migraines in children may follow a different pattern from the one they do in adults. For one, they tend to be shorter. Also, children often suffer from abdominal pain and diarrhea as well as the typical adult symptoms, such as nausea and sensitivity to light. The nausea often is severe in children and comes on early in the migraine. And although adult migraines are usually concentrated on one side of the head, children often experience pain on both sides.

Tension headaches in children, on the other hand, tend to resemble tension headaches in adults. If the headaches are severe and recurring, they are likely to be migraines and are treated as such because distinguishing between a severe tension headache and a mild migraine is very difficult, if not impossible.

If your child is getting severe or regular headaches, it is important to consult a doctor to rule out any physiological problems. About one in twenty children is not suffering from a tension or migraine headache, but from a neurological illness, infection, or other potentially serious medical condition. Assuming that's not the case, the next step is to try to relieve the pain with nondrug strategies and over-the-counter medications, and, if possible, to identify and avoid headache triggers.

NONDRUG STRATEGIES TO PREVENT
HEADACHES IN CHILDREN

Before we discuss how to avoid tension headaches and migraines — the two most common types of headaches in children — consider that some headaches in children are caused by eyestrain (too much TV or time before a computer monitor, a need for prescriptive eyeglasses) or an injury to the head. These factors may be involved when your child complains of headaches.

IDENTIFYING AND AVOIDING TRIGGERS can be very effective in warding off migraines in children. These factors include certain foods, too little sleep, smoke and other fumes, weather changes, fatigue, stress, bright lights, hunger, heavy exercise, travel, and so on. We explore these triggers in detail in Chapter 4. In addition to the foods listed there, high-sugar and high-salt foods are also potential triggers in children. Restricting what your child eats can be difficult, especially if you need to eliminate favorite foods. Try to enlist your child's cooperation and experiment. He can either stop eating all the possible trigger foods at once, or a few at a time (the most common or likely suspects), adding them back one by one. Put together a chart and a calendar with your child; the more active your child is in maintaining these tools, the more cooperative he will tend to be.

RELAXATION AND BIOFEEDBACK techniques can be very effective with children as young as seven or eight who can learn the simple breathing and imaging techniques to deal with stress that could be triggering headaches. Children nine and older can learn the more complex adult techniques described in Chapter 2. Because children are sensitive to stress, consider whether your child's routine is too hectic. Medication in children should be minimal, so it is extremely important to explore these techniques fully. They can be very effective yet are tragically underused.

PEER GROUPS OR INDIVIDUAL COUNSELING is especially useful for adolescents and their parents. Many children and adolescents who get severe headaches drive themselves hard, insist on perfection, participate in many activities, are completely stressed out and prone to depression, and need to explore and share these issues with peers in a similar situation or with a psychotherapist. Talk to your child's doctor or guidance counselor. If there is not an appropriate group already in your area, think about starting one.

RELIEVING HEADACHES IN CHILDREN UNDER AGE ELEVEN

Once headaches start, the fairly simple methods that follow can relieve the vast majority. If the child is older than eleven, the strategies shift toward the management techniques for adults. We'll address specific adolescent concerns later in this chapter.

At the first sign of a headache, either migraine or tension, get your child comfortable in a dark, quiet room and apply ice to his head. Consult with his doctor about experimenting with limited amounts of acetaminophen or ibuprofen and perhaps some caffeine.

FIRST-LINE MEDICATIONS FOR RELIEVING HEADACHES IN CHILDREN

1. ACETAMINOPHEN

Acetaminophen, the medication used in Tylenol, is well tolerated, safe, and has few side effects, but it is not as effective as ibuprofen or aspirin. Because it is safe, however, acetaminophen is usually the first medication children should try. Giving the child some caffeine, such as cola, can enhance the drug's effectiveness. Chewable tablets, liquid, and suppository forms are available.

ASPIRIN-FREE EXCEDRIN combines acetaminophen with 65 mg of caffeine and is more useful for migraine than for daily headache. Children often need to be at least nine to tolerate this dose of caffeine.

TYPICAL DOSE: When calculating by weight, the dose is approximately 3 to 5 mg per pound (5 to 10 mg per kg) every two to four hours (maximum per day of 15 or 20 mg per pound or 30 or 40 mg per kg). Three doses in twenty-four hours at most.

By age, rather than weight, typical doses are 240 mg per dose for four- and five-year-olds, 320 mg per dose for six- to eight-year-olds, 400 mg for nine- and ten-year-olds, and 480 mg per dose for eleven-year-olds. Three doses per twenty-four hours should be the maximum. If your child needs more than one dose a day, *every day*, however, consider preventive medication.

Acetaminophen is available in many forms, including chewable tablets in 80, 120, and 160 mg; regular (nonchewable) tablets in 325, 500, and 650 mg; capsules in 325 or 500 mg; and syrup in concentrations of 80, 120, 160, and 325 mg per teaspoon. There is also a Tylenol Extra-Strength liquid with 500 mg per three teaspoons.

Suppositories are available in strengths of 120, 125, 325, 600, and 650 mg. Finally, there is a fizzy antacid with buffered acetaminophen that contains 325 mg per three-quarters of a cap, as well as sodium bicarbonate and citric acid.

SIDE EFFECTS: Rare. Occasional fatigue.

2. IBUPROFEN

Ibuprofen is the generic chemical used in Advil, Motrin, and Nuprin, among others. It is more effective for migraines and tension headaches than acetaminophen but poses a greater risk of causing gastrointestinal upset, nausea, fatigue, and dizziness. Nevertheless, it is generally well tolerated. Again, giving your child caffeine in some form can enhance the drug's effectiveness. Liquid Advil is useful for younger children.

TYPICAL DOSE: Ages four to five, 100 mg (one teaspoon of the Children's Advil liquid) every three to four hours, as needed; ages six to eight, 100 to 150 mg (one to one and a half teaspoons) every three to four hours, as needed; ages nine to ten, 150 to 200 mg per dose; ages eleven to twelve, 200 to 400 mg per dose. Three doses per day at most. Maximum daily dose is 15 mg per pound (30 mg per kg) per day.

3. CAFFEINE

Caffeine can be used by itself (in a cola drink or in pill form) or with acetaminophen or ibuprofen. It can help either a tension or a migraine headache. When used in limited amounts, its side effects are minimal.

PRESCRIPTION ABORTIVE MEDICATIONS

When the simpler combinations of acetaminophen, ibuprofen, and caffeine aren't powerful enough to help your child, you'll probably need to identify with your child's doctor a stronger abortive medication to relieve a headache in progress. In the vast majority of cases with children, a good abortive is all that you'll need. However, if the abortive needs to be used more than three times a week or the headaches are sporadic but severe (and therefore usually considered migraines), the doctor may recommend a preventive medication.

As we discuss in other chapters, many medications helpful for headache have not received specific approval from the FDA for headache or for children. You should fully understand the risks, side effects, and problems associated with any medication before you give it to your child. Check a medication reference book or the package insert. Any discussion of medications here is for information, not a suggestion for use. Only a physician who knows your child's individual situation can make an informed recommendation.

If you know from experience that you will want to give the child an abortive medication if a headache starts, do so as early as possible to make it most effective. If the child is nauseated, either wait for the nausea to subside or for the child to vomit, and then use the abortive medication, or consider an antinausea medication. Rectal suppositories for combating nausea are more effective than oral medication and more useful when oral medications are not well tolerated; many children, however, feel too embarrassed to use them. Remember also that almost all of the medications listed in this chapter may be formulated by pharmacists into flavored lozenges for children who cannot swallow pills or are too nauseated to swallow medication.

If your child is ten or younger and a combination of caffeine, acetaminophen, and ibuprofen doesn't work, your doctor will probably recommend one of these medications.

FIRST-LINE MEDICATIONS FOR TREATING HEADACHES IN CHILDREN

1. NAPROXEN (ALEVE, NAPROSYN, ANAPROX)

More effective than acetaminophen or ibuprofen, naproxen does often cause temporary gastrointestinal distress. Sedation also occasionally occurs. Its liquid form can be particularly useful for children. Having a small amount of caffeine with naproxen can usually enhance its effectiveness. A lower-dose naproxen tablet (Aleve) is available over the counter but should be used only under a doctor's supervision, as is true for all prescription medications.

If used daily, kidney and liver functions need be monitored.

TYPICAL DOSE: For a fifty-pound child, one teaspoon, or 125 mg, to start; may be repeated once per day. For an eighty-five-pound child, one to one and a half teaspoons, or 125 to about 185 mg per dose; may be repeated once only. For a child one hundred pounds or more, 275 mg of Anaprox or 250 mg of naproxen or 220 mg of Aleve.

2. MIDRIN

Usually Midrin is recommended when neither the over-the-counter medications nor naproxen works well. This medication, available in capsule form, consists of acetaminophen, a mild vasoconstrictor (isometheptene mucate), and a nonaddicting sedative (dichloralphenazone). The large capsules may be taken apart and emptied into applesauce or juice (the capsule shell itself does not need to be swallowed). Midrin tends to be reasonably effective and may be used in children as young as age seven. See Chapter 5 for more details.

TYPICAL DOSE: For ages seven and eight, a quarter or half capsule, repeated every two hours if necessary but limited to two full capsules in one day. For ages nine and ten, a half or whole capsule, repeated if necessary at two-hour intervals, three in one day at the most.

SIDE EFFECTS: Sedation and lightheadedness, occasional stomach upset.

If these first-line medications are ineffective or inappropriate for your child, the doctor may then recommend:

SECOND-LINE MEDICATIONS FOR
TREATING HEADACHES IN CHILDREN

1. BUTALBITAL COMPOUNDS

These medications are generally well tolerated and extremely effective. The butalbital is a sedative, which in most cases is useful to help the child sleep away the headache.

Fiorinal (which contains aspirin) is more effective than Esgic or Fioricet (which contains acetaminophen and caffeine), which, in turn, is more effective than Phrenilin (acetaminophen but no caffeine). See Chapter 5 for more information.

• **FIORINAL**

Fiorinal contains 50 mg of the short-acting sedative butalbital, 325 mg of aspirin, and 40 mg of caffeine, which helps offset the sedative. The tablets may be cut in half for children. Because of the aspirin component, this medication must be used with caution to avoid the risk of Reye's syndrome, a disease of the brain, marked by fever, vomiting, and swelling of the kidneys and brain.

TYPICAL DOSE: For ages seven and eight, half a tablet, which may be repeated within an hour or two, but daily maximum should be no more than one tablet per day. For ages nine and ten, a half or whole tablet, which may be repeated in three hours, with a maximum of two tablets in one day.

SIDE EFFECTS: Fatigue and sometimes nervousness; nausea or gastrointestinal pain from the aspirin; lightheadedness, dizziness, or euphoria from the butalbital.

- **ESGIC, FIORICET**

These medications, which are identical except that Esgic is available in capsule or pill form and Fioricet only in pill form, are less effective than Fiorinal but better tolerated because they contain acetaminophen rather than aspirin. They consist of 50 mg of butalbital, 325 mg of acetaminophen, and 40 mg of caffeine. Since the brand name medications are usually more effective the generic is best avoided.

TYPICAL DOSE: Same as for Fiorinal.

SIDE EFFECTS: Fatigue, occasional nervousness; nausea but less so than with Fiorinal. Lightheadedness, dizziness, and euphoria may occur.

- **PHRENILIN**

Phrenilin (50 mg of butalbital and 325 mg of acetaminophen) is the same as Esgic but has no caffeine. It is particularly helpful for children who cannot take caffeine or aspirin.

TYPICAL DOSE: Same as for Fiorinal.

SIDE EFFECTS: Usually mild, though sedation is very common. Lightheadedness, dizziness, and euphoria may occur.

2. ASPIRIN

Although aspirin is quite effective and well tolerated, it is not a first choice because of the fear, founded or unfounded, of Reye's syndrome. However, unless a child has chicken pox or the flu with fever, aspirin is a safe bet. Nevertheless, many parents are reluctant to use aspirin in any situation.

Taking aspirin with caffeinated soda can relieve pain even more.

TYPICAL DOSE: For ages six to eight: 325 mg three times a day. For ages nine to ten: 400 mg three times a day, at most. Children's aspirin is available in 65, 75, and 81 mg tablets, and in 81 mg chewable tablets. Aspergum (chewing gum) has 227.5 mg each. Standard aspirin is 325 mg per tablet.

SIDE EFFECTS: Gastrointestinal upset.

When none of the first- or second-line medications is useful and your child continues to suffer from severe, prolonged headaches, which will probably be diagnosed as migraines, your doctor may recommend Prednisone or DHE. When prescribed for children, these drugs are used in very limited doses and for very short periods of time. Also remember that you can ask a pharmacist to formulate these medications into lozenges.

THIRD-LINE MEDICATIONS FOR TREATING HEADACHES IN CHILDREN

1. PREDNISONE

Prednisone becomes useful when your child is enduring a prolonged pattern of migraines which has been resistant to other medications. It should be able to break the painful cycle. Occasionally, small doses of Decadron, a corticosteroid (see Chapter 5), may be used instead.

TYPICAL DOSE: Usually 10 mg by mouth twice a day, with food, as needed, for one or two days only; 40 mg total per migraine. If the headache is relieved with smaller doses, then medication should be stopped.

SIDE EFFECTS: In these small doses, side effects are minimal. Anxiety or gastrointestinal upset are the most common. Fatigue, insomnia, and dizziness may also occur.

2. DHE

Although children do not tend to tolerate DHE well, it is sometimes the only medication that effectively relieves a severe and prolonged migraine. Administering this medication intravenously is preferred because it is more effective, less painful, and better tolerated by children than intramuscular injections.

As adults do, children should take an antinausea medication, trimethobenzamide (Tigan) or promethazine (Phenergan) before the injection.

TYPICAL DOSE: One-time dose of 0.3 to 0.5 mg intravenously. When the migraine is severe and resistant to other therapies, a second dose may be given.

SIDE EFFECTS: Nausea, lightheadedness, a feeling of heat about the head, muscle contraction headaches, and leg cramps may occur.

See Chapter 5 for a detailed discussion of this medication.

ANTINAUSEA MEDICATIONS FOR CHILDREN

As we mentioned previously, many children get nauseated with a migraine, especially early in the headache. It is usually better to let children throw up and then give them an abortive medication to ease the pain. If they can't keep the medication down, then try an antinausea medication. Unfortunately, there sometimes is little choice but to use a suppository (although a pharmacist may be able to formulate a flavored lozenge for you). These medications not only ease nausea, but in some cases, such as with promethazine, they will sedate the child, thereby helping to relieve the migraine.

Trimethobenzamide (Tigan) or promethazine (Phenergan) are the most commonly prescribed antinausea medications for children. They are detailed in Chapter 5. Other, more effective medications, such as prochlorperazine (Compazine) cause more disturbing side effects, such as anxiety, in children.

1. TRIMETHOBENZAMIDE (TIGAN)

Tigan is extremely well tolerated, which is why it is so commonly used in children.

TYPICAL DOSE: 100 to 200 mg every four hours as needed

to relieve nausea. Available in capsules, suppositories, syrups, and injections, or may be formulated as a flavored lozenge by a compounding pharmacist.

SIDE EFFECTS: Fatigue. Low blood pressure (hypotension), confusion, blurred vision, disorientation, muscle cramps, and dizziness occasionally occur.

2. PROMETHAZINE (PHENERGAN)

Phenergan is also well tolerated and often causes sedation, which may be desired.

TYPICAL DOSE: 12.5 to 25 mg per dose, or 0.15 to 0.25 per pound (0.25 to 0.5 mg per kg per dose), which may be repeated if necessary; three doses per day is the usual maximum. Available in tablets, syrup, suppositories, or injection. Flavored oral lozenges may be formulated by a compounding pharmacist.

SIDE EFFECTS: Sedation, which is helpful for relieving pain by inducing sleep. Low blood pressure (hypotension), blurred vision, disorientation, and dizziness may occur but are not common.

PREVENTING HEADACHES IN
CHILDREN UNDER AGE ELEVEN

If biofeedback and nonmedication therapies have been earnestly tried to no avail and your child is taking an abortive medication frequently and still getting more than three or four moderate to severe migraines in a typical month, your doctor may recommend preventive medication.

When considering a preventive, be prepared to use it daily and expect the possibility of some side effects as well as the potential need to change medications if one doesn't prove effective or causes severe side effects. Preventive medication in children and adolescents should be kept to a minimum and stopped periodically. As with adults, the goal is to return to abortive medications exclusively if possible.

For children younger than age eleven, the medications used to prevent migraines tend to be the same as for chronic (tension) daily headache, so they are not separated out here unless indicated.

PRESCRIPTION MEDICATIONS FOR PREVENTING HEADACHES IN CHILDREN

1. CYPROHEPTADINE (PERIACTIN)

This medication, an antihistamine often prescribed for allergies, also influences serotonin. It is inexpensive and safe, though it is not always the most effective choice. It tends to be most useful for children ten years old and younger. Because it may be taken just once a day and in liquid form, it can be quite convenient.

TYPICAL DOSE: 4 mg per day, tablet or liquid, taken at night; doses may be gradually increased to as high as 12 mg, as needed. Larger doses are split for twice-a-day dosing.

SIDE EFFECTS: Fatigue and weight gain due to increased appetite.

2. NSAIDs (IBUPROFEN, NAPROXEN)

A daily anti-inflammatory can be very effective in preventing headaches and may be preferred to the other preventives because it has no effect on energy level, sedation, or cognitive functions (memory or concentration problems). Its doses should be kept to a minimum and, with blood tests performed periodically, long-term use can be quite safe. NSAIDs have been used safely for years, for example, for juvenile rheumatoid arthritis in doses much higher than used for headaches.

TYPICAL DOSE: For ibuprofen, at age five, half a teaspoon of the 100 mg syrup, or 50 mg per day. At ages six to eight, the dose is half to one teaspoon, or 50 to 100 mg per day.

At ages nine to ten, the dose increases to one or two teaspoons, or 100 to 200 mg per day.

Naproxen doses are calculated by weight, half to one teaspoon daily. One teaspoon is equal to half of the 250 mg pill. See "First-Line Medications for Treating Headaches in Children" for more details.

3. PROPRANOLOL (INDERAL)

This beta-blocker that prevents blood vessel dilation is quite effective for migraines but only occasionally effective for daily headaches. It is very well tolerated but should not be taken by asthmatic children.

TYPICAL DOSE: 0.5 to 1.5 mg per pound per day (or 1 to 3 mg per kg per day), starting with a low dose and increasing it if necessary. The long-acting capsule cannot be divided.

SIDE EFFECTS: Fatigue and lower abdominal upset are fairly common. Less common is a decrease in heart rate and blood pressure, with a corresponding decrease in stamina. Memory or concentration difficulties, dizziness, and lightheadedness may occur.

4. ANTIDEPRESSANTS

Because of their effects on serotonin, antidepressants, such as amitriptyline (Elavil) or nortriptyline (Pamelor, Aventyl), are a first-choice medication for moderate to severe chronic daily headaches. They are usually not prescribed for migraines, however, until cyproheptadine, and the NSAIDs have been tried.

Amitriptyline and nortriptyline are similar medications, except that amitriptyline is less expensive and tends to be somewhat more effective. Nortriptyline, however, tends to have fewer side effects. For fuller discussion of amitriptyline and nortriptyline, see Chapters 6 and 9 on preventive medications for migraines and tension headaches in adults.

TYPICAL DOSE: 10 mg to start, usually at night, increased

if necessary to 25 or 50 mg (occasionally up to 75 or 100 mg). The average dose in this age range is 25 mg.

SIDE EFFECTS: Fatigue, sedation, anxiety, weight gain, a dry mouth, and dizziness; insomnia and memory or concentration difficulties may follow; occasional rapid heartbeat and blurred vision.

RELIEVING HEADACHES IN ADOLESCENTS OVER AGE ELEVEN

Encourage your adolescent to use biofeedback or relaxation therapies as much as possible. Unfortunately, though, many teens don't stick with the regimens, or their headaches are too painful for these relaxation methods to work. Although most adolescents don't need preventive medication, many do need abortive medication to relieve a headache in progress. During periods of severe or frequent headaches, however, daily preventive medication may be necessary on a temporary basis. Preventive medication may also be called for if your teen chases after headaches all day with abortive medications, which can trigger rebound headaches.

Tension and migraine headaches are treated similarly in teens, except that migraine sufferers often need an antinausea medication as well. Teens take the same medications as children do, except that they may use aspirin more readily and may be able to tolerate some stronger medications. Because we have detailed all these medications elsewhere, we simply list them here to indicate the order in which they are usually prescribed for adolescents, as well as their most prominent features and the most typical doses for teenagers. These doses tend to be the same as the low-range doses for adults. As always, these medications should be taken with food.

FIRST-LINE MEDICATIONS FOR TREATING HEADACHES IN ADOLESCENTS

1. ACETAMINOPHEN
Best tolerated, least effective. Typical dose: 325 to 650 mg every four to six hours, as needed.

2. IBUPROFEN
More effective than acetaminophen but causes more side effects, especially stomach upset. Typical dose: 200 or 400 mg every four to six hours, as needed. Take with food.

3. NAPROXEN (ALEVE, NAPROSYN, ANAPROX)
Widely used in adolescents, but stomach upset is common. Typical dose: For Aleve, 220-mg tablet every eight hours; for Naprosyn, 250-mg pill every 8 hours, as needed, higher doses in older adolescents; and for Anaprox, 275-mg pill taken with the same frequency as Naprosyn.

4. ASPIRIN, ASPIRIN-FREE EXCEDRIN, ANACIN, EXCEDRIN EXTRA-STRENGTH
- **ASPIRIN**
  Typical dose: 325 mg every four to six hours, as needed.
- **ASPIRIN-FREE EXCEDRIN**
  Typical dose: one tablet every four to six hours, as needed.
- **ANACIN (ASPIRIN AND CAFFEINE)**
  Stomach upset is common and nervousness may occur. Typical dose: one Anacin tablet every four to six hours, as needed.
- **EXCEDRIN EXTRA-STRENGTH (ACETAMINOPHEN, ASPIRIN, AND CAFFEINE)**
  Most effective medication in this group but causes more side effects, such as rebound headaches, gastrointestinal upset, and nervousness. Typical dose: One tablet every four to six hours, as needed.

**5. NORGESIC FORTE (ASPIRIN, CAFFEINE, AND AN ANTI-
HISTAMINE, ORPHENADRINE CITRATE, WITH MUSCLE RE-
LAXANT PROPERTIES)**

Strong but nonaddicting. Typical dose: Half to one pill every
three to four hours, as needed. Side effects include nervousness,
drowsiness, and a dry mouth.

SECOND-LINE MEDICATIONS FOR
TREATING HEADACHES IN ADOLESCENTS

When the first-line medications don't work, your teen's doctor
will probably then recommend one of these choices:

1. MIDRIN

Especially good for migraines. Typical dose: One capsule, repeated every two hours if needed; daily maximum dose is four
or five tablets.

**2. BUTALBITAL COMPOUNDS (FIORINAL, FIORICET, ESGIC,
PHRENILIN)**

Habit-forming. Typical dose: Varies by medication but typically
between the child and adult doses.

PREVENTING HEADACHES IN ADOLESCENTS
OVER AGE ELEVEN

As with adults, psychotherapy or biofeedback can help some
adolescents a great deal. But others who chase pain frequently
with abortive medications, which can cause rebound headaches,
will need a daily preventive for moderate or severe headaches.

Since patterns of tension and migraine headaches are more
prominent in teenagers than in younger children, the treatments
do differ somewhat, as they do in adults. One major differ-

ence, however, is that as children become adolescents the anti-inflammatories are a first-choice preventive for chronic daily headaches because they are so well tolerated by this age group. Again, these medications are detailed elsewhere, and we list them here in order of preference. The doses fall between that of those recommended for children and adults and will vary depending upon your teen's age and weight.

MEDICATIONS FOR PREVENTING TENSION HEADACHES IN ADOLESCENTS

1. ANTI-INFLAMMATORIES
IBUPROFEN AND NAPROXEN
Very well tolerated and often effective, though they may cause stomach upset.

2. ANTIDEPRESSANTS
NORTRIPTYLINE (PAMELOR, AVENTYL), PROTRIPTYLINE (VIVACTIL), AMITRIPTYLINE (ELAVIL)
These drugs are the most effective preventives for migraines and daily headaches, but they cause more side effects (memory and concentration problems, a dry mouth, and dizziness are common) than the anti-inflammatories. Usually well tolerated in low doses and safe for long-term use.

3. BETA-BLOCKERS
PROPRANOLOL (INDERAL), NADOLOL (CORGARD)
Occasionally effective for daily tension headaches, but generally more useful with migraines. They can affect your child's tolerance to exercise, which is a problem in this age range. Cognitive side effects and sedation also limit the utility of beta-blockers.

MEDICATIONS FOR PREVENTING MIGRAINES
IN ADOLESCENTS

If your adolescent is getting more than four migraines a month or if his migraines are very severe and fairly regular, his doctor will probably recommend preventive therapy. Sometimes preventive medication is even recommended for as little as one or two migraines per month if they are very severe and disruptive. The goal, as always, is to decrease frequency or severity by at least 70 percent, with as little medication as possible.

The first choices for preventing migraines in adolescents, in order of preference, are:

1. **Anti-inflammatories** are the first choices, as they are for tension headaches.
2. **Verapamil (Isoptin, Calan, Verelan)** is the next choice. Generally well tolerated, but constipation is common.
3. **Tricyclic antidepressants** are highly effective. Tricyclics are the older antidepressants, such as amitriptyline, as opposed to the newer ones, like Prozac.
4. **Beta-blockers.** See the previous list, as well as details in other chapters on preventive medications.

If these first-line drugs prove ineffective or inappropriate, your doctor may suggest one of the following second-line choices:

1. **Valproate (Depakote)** is an antiseizure medication that often causes nausea, stomach pains, and sedation.
2. **Fluoxetine (Prozac)** is not appropriate for younger adolescents. It may cause anxiety, nausea, or insomnia.
3. **Combining two of the first- or second-line medications**

The third-line choices for preventing migraines in teens are:

1. **Phenelzine (Nardil),** an MAO inhibitor

2. Intravenous DHE

Please refer to previous chapters for details on all these medications.

CASE STUDIES

Here are some fairly typical cases among children and adolescents with migraines or tension headaches.

MEREDITH

INITIAL VISIT: Meredith is a nine-year-old with a history of migraines, twice a month, ever since she was six. The migraines last five hours, with a severe but short bout of nausea. Undersleeping and chocolate are the only consistent triggers for Meredith's migraines. She also gets tension headaches, which occur three or four times a week and tend to worsen with stress. They usually occur toward the end of the school day and decrease in the summer.

Meredith's doctor teaches her basic deep-breathing–relaxation techniques, as age nine is a good time to try these methods. Meredith learns how to apply reusable ice packs to her head. Tylenol has been effective for her tension headaches, and she takes three or four chewable Tylenol tablets a week. Caffeine, in Coke or Pepsi, also helps. Meredith learns all of the usual migraine avoidance techniques, such as eating a diet absent of trigger foods and wearing dark sunglasses on bright days. The first goal to try to avoid more medication.

WEEK 2: Meredith's mother reports that the deep-breathing–relaxation techniques are helping to relieve the tension headaches, but Meredith is still getting migraines. The doctor writes a prescription for liquid ibuprofen (Children's Advil), as Meredith has a difficult time swallowing tablets.

WEEK 4: The ibuprofen helps relieve the migraine pain

somewhat but increases her nausea. Meredith receives a prescription for liquid promethazine (Phenergan) for the nausea.

WEEK 16: The ibuprofen is no longer effective, but the liquid Phenergan helps relieve the nausea. Meredith's doctor prescribes Midrin for the migraine pain and shows Meredith and her mom how to pull apart the capsule and put the powder in juice or applesauce.

WEEK 19: The Phenergan and Midrin are sedating Meredith but are helping to reduce the pain by about 80 percent. Meredith wishes to try a medication that won't make her so sleepy. The Midrin is discontinued, and Meredith tries liquid Naprosyn, an anti-inflammatory similar to ibuprofen, instead.

WEEK 22: The Naprosyn helps the pain about 60 percent and does not sedate Meredith. Although it increases her nausea, the Phenergan is controlling it. The plan is now for Meredith to use the Phenergan-Naprosyn combination if she's in school with pain, but if she's at home with a migraine she'll use Phenergan with Midrin, which is more effective but puts her to sleep. Such a choice is not unusual for headache patients. They learn to use different medications in different situations.

THE FUTURE: If Meredith needs a change of medication, her doctor may prescribe a pure migraine medication, such as ergotamine (Cafergot) or dihydroergotamine (DHE). As of this writing, sumatriptan (Imitrex) is not usually given to children. Butalbital medications, such as Fiorinal, Fioricet, Esgic, or Phrenilin, may also be helpful for Meredith at some point. Sedatives, such as diazepam (Valium), or narcotics, such as codeine, occasionally are useful in children of Meredith's age but are not generally used until other alternatives have been exhausted.

MICHAEL

INITIAL VISIT: Michael, a ten-year-old boy, has had monthly migraines since he was eight. Six months ago, he started to get moderately severe daily headaches. The migraines are also moderate to severe, last eight hours, and usually stop when he falls asleep. Michael vomits early in the migraine and then feels better. He becomes carsick easily, which is common among children with migraines. There is a strong family history of migraines, as both his mother and father have had migraines in the past. Michael does well in school and is a hard-driving perfectionist.

Acetaminophen or ibuprofen is only slightly effective for Michael's migraines. Caffeinated soft drinks do help to some degree. For the monthly migraine, Michael's doctor prescribes Midrin. Michael empties the contents of the large capsule into applesauce. He puts ice packs on his head as well.

The chronic daily headaches are more of a burden to Michael than the migraines. They last most of the day, every day. Occasionally, we find that children with headaches are "overprogrammed" and under too much stress. While the headaches are worse with stress, they are also present when Michael is relaxed and on vacation. He and the doctor practice deep-breathing and relaxation techniques. After some discussion with Michael's parents, they decide to decrease his activities so that he does not have a planned activity day after day.

WEEK 2: The Midrin helps Michael's migraine, as do the ice packs, but makes him sedated and lightheaded. His doctor prescribes Cafergot instead of Midrin to help relieve any migraine. His daily headaches remain as bad as ever, and the doctor prescribes naproxen as a preventive medication, 250 mg per day.

WEEK 4: Michael's mother calls to say that the naproxen is working well to prevent the daily headaches, but that Michael had a migraine yesterday and the Cafergot made him very sick. The doctor calls in a prescription to the pharmacy for Fioricet (acetaminophen, caffeine, and the mild sedative butalbital) to replace the Cafergot.

FOUR MONTHS LATER: Michael comes in and reports that he has felt better for several months, but his daily headaches are back. Evidently, the naproxen has lost its effectiveness. The doctor prescribes a low dose of amitriptyline (Elavil), 10 mg, to be taken at night.

WEEK 1: Michael's mother calls to say the medication seems to have no effect. The dose is raised to 25 mg.

WEEK 2: Michael's mother calls to say that the daily headaches have eased somewhat, but she would like to try a higher dose. The amitriptyline dose is raised to 50 mg.

WEEK 4: Michael's daily headaches have vastly improved, but Michael is tired, with a dry mouth. His dose is lowered to 35 mg.

TWO MONTHS LATER: Michael comes in for a checkup, and his mother reports that the side effects of the Elavil have abated. The daily headaches are 50 to 70 percent improved.

THE FUTURE: The goal with children is to minimize medication yet alleviate the headaches. Because 35 mg of amitriptyline appears to be the highest dose that Michael can tolerate, if the headaches get worse, he should consider nortriptyline (Pamelor or Aventyl), a milder form of amitriptyline. While not quite as effective as amitriptyline, the nortriptyline often produces milder side effects. A beta-blocker such as propranolol (Inderal), may help. If the headaches remain very much improved, the daily preventive medication should be discontinued periodically to assess whether it is still necessary. Many children go off and on daily preventive medication depending on the severity of their headaches. In a boy such as Michael, there is a 50 percent chance that he will outgrow the headaches by age twenty.

RICHARD

INITIAL VISIT: Richard, a seventeen-year-old high school student, has a five-year history of migraines once a month; more recently, the headaches have increased to twice a month. He also gets very mild, frequent tension headaches, but they do not bother him. The migraines are very severe, lasting sixteen to twenty-four hours, with mild nausea. All of the over-the-counter medications have been ineffective. Richard's mother and sister both have had headaches. Richard is usually a good student, but this semester he has started to stay home from school more frequently and his grades have fallen.

He and his doctor discuss diet, relaxation techniques, and the other nonmedication strategies. Richard has been using marijuana and alcohol at least three times a week. He agrees to stop, as the drugs may be responsible for worsening his headache situation. Because of his recent history of missing classes and doing poorly in school, his doctor suggests a consultation with a psychotherapist. Age seventeen is a difficult time for many adolescents, who may experience hidden stresses and depressions. Using headaches to avoid classes may also be a symptom of school phobia, which Richard needs to address with a therapist.

WEEK 4: Richard is seeing a therapist and reports that relaxation techniques have helped his milder headaches, but that the migraines persist. He receives a prescription for Midrin as an abortive medication to relieve the pain once it starts. His migraines do not occur frequently enough to justify the use of a daily preventive approach.

WEEK 6: Richard calls to say that the Midrin is mildly effective but makes him very drowsy. The doctor switches his prescription to ergotamine (Cafergot).

WEEK 8: Richard calls to say that Cafergot makes him very nauseated. The doctor now prescribes Anaprox, an anti-inflammatory, to be taken with Reglan, a mild antinausea medication. This is a nonaddicting, first-line medication tactic.

THREE MONTHS LATER: Richard reports the medications in combination are working well.

THREE MONTHS LATER: Richard reports that the Anaprox and Reglan are no longer effective. His doctor prescribes DHE (dihydroergotamine) nasal spray. DHE is safe, nonaddicting, and can actually abort a headache, not simply cover the pain. Richard calls after his next migraine to say it is effective.

THREE MONTHS LATER: Richard phones to report that the DHE no longer works. Richard's doctor does not want to prescribe the butalbital medications (Fiorinal, Esgic, Phrenilin, Axotal) for Richard. These drugs are mildly habit-forming, and Richard has a history of overusing alcohol and marijuana. Instead, his physician explains how to self-inject sumatriptan (Imitrex). Now eighteen years old, Richard is not afraid of injections.

WEEK 6: Richard reports that the Imitrex is working well, although he experiences twenty minutes of mild nausea after the injection, as well as chest pressure and tingling in his arms. All of these side effects, however, go away easily and the headache dissipates within one hour. Richard remains slightly fatigued but is able to function well the rest of the day. He decides that he will take these injections with him as he goes away to college.

THE FUTURE: Other possibilities for Richard include oral sumatriptan (Imitrex pills, which are not as effective but are more convenient than the injections), Cafergot PB suppositories, DHE injections, or, as a last resort, a butalbital compound or narcotic analgesic.

12

. . . .

LESS COMMON HEADACHES AND TREATMENTS

IN THIS CHAPTER, we'll look at other kinds of headaches that are actually less common, though some are very well known, such as sinus headaches and sexual headaches. In most cases, these headaches are named for their triggers and are similar to the types of headaches we have discussed so far. Nevertheless, many people identify their headache by its triggers, so it's useful to address each one separately.

POST-TRAUMATIC HEADACHE

Headaches are very common after a rear-end car accident, whether or not your head or neck was injured in the collision. This is particularly true if you have suffered from headaches before. Usually these headaches develop within hours or days of the accident, although occasionally they may begin months later. In most cases, the headaches will taper off within a few days to several weeks. However, even minor accidents can produce very severe, long-lasting headaches of up to a year or more.

Post-traumatic headaches are usually either tension-type headaches — daily or episodic — or more severe migraine-type headaches, or both. Neck and back-of-the-head pain are also very common. Typical symptoms that may accompany these headaches are poor concentration, becoming easily angered or frustrated, sensitivity to noise or bright lights, depression, dizziness, ringing in the ears, memory problems, fatigue, insomnia, lack of motivation, lessening sexual drive, nervousness or anxiety, irritability, and decreased ability to comprehend complex issues.

When someone is suffering from these symptoms, it's not uncommon for family members and coworkers to think that person is exaggerating his pain or malingering. Yet these headaches and symptoms are very real, and the head pain, anxiety, insomnia, and difficulty concentrating can be disabling and interfere with home or work responsibilities. A vicious cycle can develop, in which the victim suffers from additional psychological stress stemming from these frustrations and difficulties.

Nevertheless, if you've been in an accident or endured some other kind of head injury that is now causing headaches (or some of the other symptoms we've listed), you should definitely consult a doctor to assess the physical injury. The doctor may suggest physical therapy, psychological counseling, relaxation training or biofeedback, medication, or a combination of these treatments.

RELIEVING POST-TRAUMATIC HEADACHES WITH MEDICATION In the first few weeks of headaches, anti-inflammatories (aspirin, ibuprofen, and naproxen) are usually recommended because they not only help with the head pain but can also help relieve any accompanying neck or back pain. If these drugs are ineffective, the doctor may recommend a next choice from the list of medications used for tension headaches and migraines, depending on which type the pain most closely resembles. Muscle relaxants like cyclobenzaprine (Flexeril) or methocarbamol (Robaxin) may also be helpful if spasms occur in the neck, but these medications may cause fatigue.

Most people with post-traumatic migraines need only abortive medications because the headaches resolve themselves over time. However, if the headaches are migraines, occur frequently, or cause you to use excessive amounts of abortive medication, a preventive strategy may be recommended.

The antidepressants, particularly amitriptyline (Elavil) or nortriptyline (Pamelor), and the beta-blockers (Inderal, Corgard) are the most commonly prescribed preventives used for post-traumatic headaches. The sedating antidepressants, particularly amitriptyline, often help relieve daily headaches, migraines, and any associated insomnia. In severe cases, both a beta-blocker and an antidepressant may be recommended. The anti-inflammatories may also be used as a preventive.

If the headaches are migraines, calcium blockers (verapamil) may be tried as a first-line therapy. Valproate (Depakote), methysergide (Sansert), fluoxetine (Prozac), and MAO inhibitors (Phenelzine) are prescribed if these initial approaches are not successful. Intravenous dihydroergotamine (DHE), given repetitively in the office or in the hospital, is very useful with severe cases and is usually used along with a daily preventive medication.

EXERCISE AND SEXUAL HEADACHES

Exercise-induced, or exertional, headaches are for the most part benign and usually last only fifteen to twenty minutes, but occasionally all day. More common in those over forty who have just recently begun an exercise program, these headaches typically occur during or just after strenuous exercise, such as weightlifting, heading a ball in soccer, jogging, aerobics, and diving. They may also occur after sex or a bad coughing spell. Lower-impact activities, such as walking, swimming, using a treadmill, and biking are much less likely to trigger an exercise-induced headache. They are equally common in women and men.

Sexual headaches (also called orgasmic cephalalgia and benign coital headaches) are a type of exertional headache and are more common in men. If you get a sexual headache and have no history of headache problems, there is a good chance you won't get another. If you do have a headache history, your risk of recurring attacks is much higher. Nevertheless, these headaches too are usually benign, although neurologic problems that become apparent with increasing head pressure (such as meningitis, subarachnoid hemorrhage, and stroke) could manifest themselves during sex. In some people, masturbation or simply assuming the position for intercourse — lying down and anticipating pain from increased blood flow into the head — can produce a headache.

A sexual headache may be mild or, more frequently, moderate to severe. Typically, it occurs just before orgasm. Stopping intercourse when the headache begins may help shorten or diminish it. On the other hand, it has recently been reported that sex can occasionally stop a migraine or cluster headache in progress.

If you get an exercise headache, see a doctor to exclude certain medical problems. Typically, exertional headaches are treated the same way as tension or migraine headaches: by applying cold to the head, lying down in a dark room, and taking a medication as described in Chapters 5 and 8. If they occur systematically, then the doctor may suggest trying these preventives:

1. Anti-inflammatories (NSAIDs), such as indomethacin (Indocin, typical dose 50 to 75 mg), naproxen (Naprosyn, Anaprox, typical dose 500 mg), ibuprofen (Motrin, typical dose 600 to 800 mg), or flurbiprofen (Ansaid, typical dose 100 to 200 mg). These drugs should be taken a half to two hours before exercising. The effective dose varies widely.

2. Propranolol (Inderal), 20 to 60 mg, taken a half to one hour before exercising. Fatigue and decreased exercise tolerance are potential problems with propranolol.

SPINAL TAP HEADACHES

About one-third of people who have spinal taps, a diagnostic procedure, get lumbar puncture headaches. Although anyone can get one, women with a history of headaches and younger, underweight people are at highest risk.

The smaller the needle used, the smaller the risk of a subsequent headache. The position you assume after the procedure, the experience of the doctor, or the amount of spinal fluid taken do *not* appear to affect the likelihood of getting such a headache. Psychological factors play a lesser role than was once thought.

Usually the headache comes on within forty-eight hours of the spinal tap, but occasionally it may not occur until two weeks afterward. The pain may be in the front or back of the head, or in the neck and shoulder area. Typically, it hurts to sit or stand, but lying down can help. The pain may be throbbing, pounding, or ache severely.

The symptoms resemble those of migraines — nausea, visual disturbances, sensitivity to light, and dizziness — but in addition, neck pain and spasm often occur. Usually the headaches resolve themselves within days to weeks, occasionally longer. Just what causes the headaches is not known for sure, though some experts believe the mechanism may be similar to that of migraines.

For most people, simply using analgesics, as described in Chapter 2, is all that's necessary until the headaches decline. Although oral caffeine may help, it's hard to consume enough to make a significant difference. If the headache persists for more than two days, your doctor may recommend an injection of caffeine. Be warned, however, that it can cause central nervous system side effects such as jitters or tremors, as well as a rapid heartbeat. Drinking at least six glasses of liquid each day may also help.

If the headache is severe and unimproving, an epidural blood patch — an injection of your own blood in the lower back, where the spinal tap was done, can be extremely effective. This is an easy procedure for an experienced physician. And if this treatment doesn't work, then standard tension headache prevention medications may be recommended, as well as a saline solution near the spinal tap puncture.

SINUS HEADACHES

Although many people think they suffer from chronic sinus headaches, chances are they are experiencing mild migraines. Very few headaches — less than 2 percent of all headaches and less than 30 percent of recurring headaches believed to be sinus headaches — actually fit into this category.

It can be exceedingly difficult to determine the course of a frontal, or facial, headache associated with nasal congestion or stuffiness. In certain seasons or during weather changes, many people with migraines do experience a stuffy frontal headache, which they mistake for a sinus headache. A combined approach, treating both the migraines and nasal congestion, may be necessary.

True sinus headaches are caused by infections and fluid build-up in the bony pockets of the upper face. This congestion causes pressure and pain. Symptoms include a runny or stuffy nose, postnasal drip, tenderness around the sinus regions of the face, and sometimes a fever. X-rays can confirm the diagnosis of sinusitis, and antibiotics are often needed to treat the infection.

Migraines, on the other hand, are far more common than true sinus headaches but are often misidentified because they also can cause pain in the sinuses. Migraine pain is caused by the dilation of blood vessels — which may occur in the face and sinus region — as well as by irritated nerves that misfire the pain signal along the head's large trigeminal nerve, with branches throughout the face and sinus. Thus, pain in the sinus region may have nothing to do with the sinuses.

If you think you have a sinus headache and decide to take an over-the-counter sinus medication, it may work because it contains caffeine, an analgesic (aspirin or acetaminophen), or a vasoconstrictor — all substances that would help a migraine. Sinus medications with decongestants, however, can make your headache worse if it is not a true sinus headache because they can raise your blood pressure and aggravate the source of your pain. Do not overuse the OTC nasal sprays. Prescription cortisone-based nasal sprays are more effective and do not produce rebound nasal stuffiness.

ALLERGY HEADACHES

Although allergies and headaches are both very common, allergies usually do not cause headaches. Both conditions may occur at the same time, but that's purely coincidental and not a matter of cause and effect. When smoke, chocolate, or red wine, for example, cause a headache, it's probably not because you are allergic to them but sensitive to their effect on blood vessels. Much more commonly, these headaches are a migraine- or a tension-type headache. A true allergy headache, caused by an immune system that misfires, occurs only occasionally. Its symptoms are very similar to hay fever: a runny nose, sneezing, watery eyes, and sometimes a sore throat, with pain usually in the front, above and below the eyes.

Of course there are food allergies, but they more typically cause nausea, vomiting, hives, wheezing, diarrhea, rashes, and itching rather than headaches. Allergies to dairy foods and wheat products (bread and pasta) are the most common. Keep a headache diary and try to distinguish between a food sensitivity and an allergy; in either case, if you can identify the food that is triggering your headaches, avoid it. Prescription nasal (cortisone-based) sprays and antihistamines occasionally help frontal headaches. However, allergy treatments usually help the allergies themselves much more than they help the related migraines.

TMJ HEADACHES AND JAW CLENCHING (BRUXISM)

While disorders of the jaw and teeth are generally overdiagnosed as a cause of headache, TMJ and clenching (bruxism) may *add* to a headache patient's pain. It can be very difficult, however, to assess accurately the extent to which someone's teeth clenching or TMJ problem is adding to a headache situation.

Some headaches are related to problems with the temporomandibular joint (TMJ), the hinge attaching the lower jaw to the skull. It is located just in front of each ear, and if you move your jaw you can feel it. When this area is sensitive to touch, especially with a dull or stabbing headache, it may be related to a disorder of the joint but may also be a migraine or tension headache. If you have trouble opening or closing your jaw all the way, or if your jaw locks, TMJ may be the problem. Usually these headaches can be relieved with the same strategies used for tension headaches (see Chapters 2 and 8). Check with a doctor or dentist if they persist. Some people clench their teeth and jaw all day or at night, leading to increased headaches. A dentist or TMJ specialist can give you a mouth bite splint to stop you from clenching.

EYESTRAIN HEADACHES

When we overuse our eyes or do not have the proper corrective lenses, we overwork the muscles around our eyes, which can cause a tension headache. A headache from eyestrain is usually a dull, frontal ache or pain behind the eyes.

Of course, the same medications that help tension headaches will relieve eyestrain headaches, but an eye exam and improved corrective lenses would probably go further in preventing them in the future! Contact lenses do not usually offer an advantage over glasses in regard to headache.

HANGOVER HEADACHES

Alcohol can cause headaches by dilating blood vessels, wreaking havoc on the blood sugar–insulin balance, causing dehydration, or introducing chemicals to which the body is sensitive.

The most effective way to treat a hangover headache is to drink as much water as possible as well as some fruit juice or to eat some honey on crackers and take two aspirin. These strategies are most effective if taken before bed and upon awakening.

ICE CREAM HEADACHES
Some people are particularly sensitive to very cold foods, such as ice cream, and coldness may trigger sudden and severe pain in the forehead, nose, temples, or cheeks. The pain usually lasts less than a minute.

TIGHT-HAT HEADACHES
As most people know, a tight hat, swimming cap, headband, or swimming goggles may cause pressure or irritate the nerves around the head and trigger a headache. In the vast majority of cases, these headaches can be simply treated with the over-the-counter analgesics described in Chapter 2.

WEEKEND AND TRAVEL HEADACHES
If you drink a lot of coffee and tea at work and don't continue this pattern on the weekend, you may get weekend headaches, which are very common. So-called caffeine withdrawal usually occurs some eighteen to thirty-six hours after the last cup of coffee or tea. Travel can wreak the same kind of havoc on your normal caffeine consumption.

These headaches can be decreased by gradually diminishing the amount of caffeine you regularly ingest so your body is not so dependent on it. Or you can be more careful in maintaining a constant level of caffeine consumption on weekends or trips.

If you get headaches after a stressful week and get a so-called Saturday morning migraine, you may need to remember to incorporate stress-reducing techniques in your week, such as physical exercise or relaxation exercises to relieve the build-up of stress and how your body holds it. These weekend stress-let-down headaches are often exceedingly difficult to treat and eliminate.

HOLIDAY HEADACHES

Some people complain that their headaches flare up during the holiday season. A combination of factors, such as the stress and frustration of getting all their holiday shopping and chores done in time, fighting crowds and traffic, and the extra strain of attending numerous social events with coworkers or relatives, is probably responsible. Also, people tend to drink more alcohol and disrupt their routines during the holidays, which can contribute to triggering headaches. Headache sufferers are particularly susceptible to disruptions in their sleeping and eating schedules. The strategies in Chapter 2 (relaxation and stress-reduction exercises and perhaps an over-the-counter pain reliever) will help keep the holidays headache-free.

AFTER-SURGERY HEADACHES

Doctors have noticed for years that patients often experience headaches after surgery. Recent studies suggest that these are actually caffeine-withdrawal headaches because of the requirement that you not eat or drink anything twelve hours prior to the surgery. Discuss this possibility with your doctor prior to surgery.

After surgery, eating and having a cup or tea or coffee and a mild over-the-counter painkiller (aspirin, acetaminophen, or ibuprofen) will probably relieve these headaches. In any case, they resolve themselves quickly.

There is anecdotal evidence that some people actually experience a *decrease* in migraines for several months after surgery. The reason for this is not known.

HEMICRANIA CONTINUA

Hemicrania continua are rare one-sided headaches of dull, throbbing, or severe pain, lasting from five to sixty minutes, three to five times per twenty-four hours. The pain is usually pulsating, with several minutes of intensely painful ice pick jabs. Men and women of all ages suffer equally, often from daily headaches. Alcohol or physical exertion often intensifies the pain. Some people may experience other symptoms similar to migraines, such as sensitivity to light and nausea.

The anti-inflammatory indomethacin is the drug of choice for hemicrania continua headaches and will relieve them in 80 percent of cases. If you can't tolerate it, or if it isn't helpful, then your doctor will probably follow the strategies for migraine prevention, suggesting amitriptyline, naproxen, or calcium blockers.

CHRONIC PAROXYSMAL HEMICRANIA (CPH)

These very rare chronic cluster headaches are treated differently from other clusters. Most common among young women between twenty-five and thirty-five, these headaches are usually one-sided and focused around an eye, temple, or the forehead. Typically, the pain lasts up to fifteen minutes and may strike anywhere from five to twenty times a day. Like other types of cluster headaches, the pain is extremely severe and often associated with a tearing eye and a stuffy or runny nose.

Such severe headaches should be assessed by a doctor to exclude the rare possibility of a tumor or an aneurysm. Once diagnosed properly, CPH headaches are almost always relieved by the anti-inflammatory indomethacin (Indocin), though the effective dose varies greatly, from as little as 25 mg to 250 mg per day. The medication should always be taken with food to avoid gastrointestinal upset. Other side effects of the medication include fatigue, lightheadedness, and mood swings. Liver and kidney blood tests need to be checked regularly to rule out any organ dysfunction.

BACK-OF-THE-HEAD PAIN

About 20 percent of migraine sufferers, as well as other headache sufferers, sometimes experience a sharp, burning, ice-pick or stabbing pain in the back of the head (occipital neuralgia). It may be accompanied by tenderness around the nerve in that area.

If severe, the pain can be relieved with a nerve-block injection of novocaine (Marcaine or Lidocaine) just under the skin. The procedure is easy, with minimal discomfort and low risk. The injection may be done once or twice but usually not more than several times a year. If effective, the pain may be relieved for weeks or months. These so-called occipital nerve blockades are also helpful for cluster headaches and their variants, such as chronic paroxysmal hemicrania. Cortisone injections in the area of the nerve are sometimes more effective than novocaine.

Back-of-the-head pain may also stem from injury, such as whiplash or shingles (herpes zoster). While antidepressants, anti-inflammatories, or the anticonvulsant carbamazepine (Tegretol) relieve such pain, many people with occipital neuralgia respond better to injections. Physical therapy to the neck occasionally is helpful.

MEDICATION-INDUCED HEADACHES

Almost all medication labels list headache as a possible side effect. Even patients who take a placebo sometimes report headaches. The *Physicians' Desk Reference* and other medication reference books often list headaches as a side effect or adverse reaction to many medications.

In susceptible individuals, almost any medication may bring on a headache, even acetaminophen, aspirin, or ibuprofen. A few medications, however, that are commonly linked to headaches, include atenolol, captropril, cimetidine, cocaine, danazol, diclofenac, nitroglycerin, oral contraceptives, and ranitidine (Zantac). In addition, calcium channel blockers, such as verapamil, can produce a chronic daily low-grade headache, and antidepressants, such as amitriptyline or fluoxetine, can increase the frequency of headaches in some people. Ironically, these medications are often prescribed for headaches because they help decrease headaches in more than half of patients who take them and aggravate headaches in only about 5 percent. Likewise, anti-inflammatories, such as ibuprofen, aspirin, and naproxen, also prescribed for headaches, occasionally aggravate a headache situation.

As we've mentioned in previous chapters, many analgesics produce rebound headaches when patients overuse them, especially medications with caffeine, which include many of the over-the-counter pain relievers. Although caffeine helps headaches when taken in small amounts, too much caffeine on a daily basis may increase headaches. Ergotamine preparations, which temporarily shrink the arteries, also often produce rebound headaches in daily dosers.

Many medications used to protect the heart or to lower blood pressure will help headaches while others induce more headaches. Nitroglycerin, for example, a medication prescribed for heart problems, often produces a headache. Antibiotics and cold preparations may also bring on headaches in some people.

Fact: Almost any medication can increase headaches in a susceptible individual.

HEADACHES CAUSED BY MEDICAL CONDITIONS
Many other factors can cause headaches, such as too much sun, high blood pressure, and a host of medical disorders.

INFECTIONS In a headache-prone person, any infection may induce headaches. A migraine sufferer with a sinus infection or the flu will probably experience a more severe and prolonged headache than a nonmigraine sufferer. Yet infections can also induce moderate to severe headaches in people who have never had a migraine or tension headache.

Meningitis (an infection involving the covering of the brain) usually produces a fever, headache, and stiff neck. HIV headache can cause severe pain, is often related to light sensitivity, and almost always occurs in conjunction with advanced infection. Any headache associated with a fever should be reported to a physician.

CIRCULATORY PROBLEMS Although most migraine sufferers experience cold feet or hands, true circulatory problems do not occur more often in headache patients than among the general population.

Stroke may produce headaches in some people, but the pain is usually minimal. Heart disease and artery disease in the arms or legs (peripheral vascular disease) does not usually cause headaches, although medications used to treat these conditions occasionally exacerbate or induce a headache.

HIGH BLOOD PRESSURE Uncontrolled high blood pressure on a moderate to severe level may cause or exacerbate headaches. *Mild* elevations in blood pressure, however, do *not* usually increase the severity or frequency of headaches. On the other hand, during the day of a migraine or cluster headache, many people will experience a rise in blood pressure.

CANCER Brain tumors may cause or aggravate headaches, but cancer in other parts of the body usually does not significantly affect head pain. Brain tumors are rare and usually coupled with progressively worse vomiting and increased head pain upon coughing and sneezing. Cancer patients should report any new neurologic symptom, such as vision changes or numbness, to a doctor. Certain medications used to treat cancer or associated medical complications may increase headaches in some people.

EYE PROBLEMS Although some severe eye problems, such as glaucoma, can cause eye pain or headache, such pain usually does not involve the eyes themselves. Nevertheless, an exam with an ophthalmologist may be very helpful to rule out the eyes as a contributing factor in headache.

EAR PROBLEMS Pain in or about the ear may represent ear disease or referred pain from the jaw joint, as in TMJ. Migraine sufferers occasionally experience a sharp, stabbing pain in or around the ear. However, migraine pain is rarely limited to the ear. When the pain around an ear is steady and constant, it is probably caused by an inner ear infection and needs a doctor's attention.

HYPOGLYCEMIA Most physicians do not believe that hypoglycemia is a real factor in headaches. However, *normal* drops in blood sugar (not *true* hypoglycemia) can produce a headache (though not necessarily a migraine) in some migraine sufferers, particularly if they haven't eaten for twelve or more hours. Diabetics who experience low blood sugar or whose diabetes is not well controlled may also get a headache, even a migraine. A glass of orange juice or a sugary food should relieve the low blood sugar and the head pain.

MISCELLANEOUS FACTORS

Some environmental contaminants may also contribute to headaches. These include benzene, carbon monoxide, formaldehyde, glutaraldehyde, hydrogen sulfide, methyl alcohol, toluene, trichloroethylene, and xylene. Other activities that may induce headaches include jet lag, an epileptic seizure, and lactation.

13

·······

MORE ALTERNATIVES

THE TECHNIQUES in this chapter, some of them unortho-
dox, can be very effective. Homeopathic remedies, for instance,
have not been scientifically researched in well-controlled studies, but some people find them useful. Whether these strategies
provide relief directly or offer a placebo is not known. The
placebo effect is real and powerful — some 35 percent of
headache sufferers report short-term relief after taking a pill
that they expect to work.

Although we do not necessarily prescribe or recommend any
of these treatments, we do think it is important to let you know
about the many options available. When appropriate, discuss
them with your physician.

TRIGGER-POINT INJECTIONS

When headaches are caused by muscle knots in the neck or
head, relief may not come easily. Trigger-point injections of
novocaine (Marcaine or Lidocaine) into the painful areas can be
very effective, perhaps offering relief for weeks or even months.
Some people, however, will find them of no benefit. Trigger
points are safe and involve an injection into the neck muscle.
Especially useful for cluster headaches, trigger-point injections
are not commonly used because of an uneven success rate. But
if you're interested, discuss this option with your doctor.

NERVE BLOCKS

Nerve blocks of novocaine are sometimes used to relieve pain in the back of the head (occipital neuralgia). For more details, please refer to Chapter 12.

HYPNOSIS AND SELF-HYPNOSIS

Unfortunately, hypnosis has not been very helpful in treating headache. Biofeedback, a form of self-hypnosis, however, has been found to be quite beneficial. See Chapter 2 for more details on biofeedback and other forms of self-hypnosis, such as imagery and relaxation techniques.

ACUPUNCTURE

Acupuncture has been used to treat headaches for more than four thousand years. While not entirely conforming to modern scientific principles, acupuncture is helpful in some circumstances and is being used increasingly in the West. It is based on the principle of reestablishing a balance between the body's yin and yang. Easterners believe that these two opposing forces, representing feminine and masculine qualities, are at work in the human body and the cosmos.

Although we don't know exactly how or why acupuncture works, acupuncturists have identified about five hundred points that are related to nerve receptors. When stimulated, pain is somehow muted. Hair-thin stainless steel needles provide stimuli to the nervous system and work most effectively when applied to an area where nerve and muscle meet. Some American scientists suggest that acupuncture temporarily stimulates nerve cells to produce the body's natural painkillers, the enkephalins and endorphins. At least one study, using rats, conducted at the University of Texas Health Sciences Center, supports this theory.

The acupuncturist may insert the needles into selected points on the body's meridians — energy considered essential to health.

He may twirl the needles, stimulate them with mild electricity, or heat them to enhance the effectiveness of treatment. Electric stimulation seems to be the most effective mode.

Studies evaluating the efficacy of acupuncture for headaches are difficult to do, considering the high placebo response. The several studies that have been conducted produced conflicting findings for headaches, and the results of long-term studies have yet to come.

Although traditional Western physicians do not wholeheartedly endorse acupuncture, many doctors believe there is little harm in trying the services of a reputable (and in some states, licensed) acupuncturist. The procedure is generally very safe; occasionally side effects may occur, such as bleeding, faintness, or infection. The American Academy of Medical Acupuncture reports that some two thousand American physicians use acupuncture in their practices.

For more information and referrals, ask your doctor or medical center. See Appendix A for specific addresses and phone numbers.

ACUPRESSURE

Acupressure involves applying circular finger pressure to some of the points that acupuncturists have identified. One acupressure point for headaches is the center of the web between your thumb and index finger. Apply pressure with the index finger from your other hand and, without lifting the finger, press in a circular motion. Other pressure points are the sides of the spine at the base of the neck.

For direct acupressure to the head, try rubbing your index fingers on the bony parts of your temples as close to the painful areas as possible, in small circles, pressing against the bone. Maintain for two minutes.

Other pressure points include the top of the ear; either side of the back of the neck at the base of the skull, where you can feel bony protrusions; and above your ears, where you can feel movement when you bite down.

TENS: TRANSCUTANEOUS ELECTRICAL NERVE STIMULATION

A TENS unit is a battery-operated device that produces a small electrical current. Its pads are usually applied to the neck and lower skull to create a tingly, or vibrating, sensation. It may relieve some pain by blocking pain transmission signals or by stimulating the production of the body's own painkillers, endorphins. While TENS has some limited usefulness for chronic pain, such as low back pain, its ability to cure headaches has been very disappointing. The relief, if any, is very temporary. Some thought has been given to developing a TENS unit that is applied to the head and affects serotonin. Such a device was tested in the 1980s, and with more research it could be helpful in alleviating chronic headaches in the future.

CHIROPRACTIC MEASURES AND PHYSICAL THERAPY

Although not useful for many people, chiropractic treatment can be very helpful for some. It may include manipulation of the spine, ultrasound, diathermy (heat on the skin), deep heat, electrical stimulation, and massage. These therapies will help some headache patients, but overall, chiropractic measures appear to benefit the neck and back to a greater degree.

Physical therapists treat head and neck pain with the same techniques (with the exception of spine manipulation). As with chiropractic measures, physical therapy usually benefits the associated neck pain more than the head pain. It is particularly useful, however, after whiplash injuries, to improve posture, to relieve neck strain, and may help headaches caused by workstation strain.

HOME REMEDIES

ICE AND HEAT PACKS Heating pads may be soothing and promote relaxation, while ice packs help reduce swelling of blood vessels. Please see Chapter 2 for more details.

SALT PACKS To relieve headache pain, *Natural Health* magazine (May–June 1993) recommends a warm salt pack applied to the back of the head. Warm salt in a dry frying pan, wrap it in a thin dish towel, and use it to rub the back of your neck.

HOT HERBAL FOOTBATHS *Natural Health* recommends an old-fashioned footbath with one tablespoon of dry mustard or ginger. Perhaps because it can be deeply relaxing, it may also provide relief.

HERBS Tea, steeped for at least thirty minutes in a closed container, may offer relief, according to *Natural Health* (May–June 1993). The magazine's recipe for a pot of tea is to combine four tablespoons of chamomile, one tablespoon of white willow bark, and one tablespoon of valerian root. According to Deepak Chopra, M.D., herbs that may help include valerian, crotalaria verrucosa, nutmeg, gotu kola, or winter cherry. Beware, however, that some herbs can be dangerous. Chaparral, germander, comfrey, mistletoe, skullcap, mate tea, yerba tea, and others have been reported to cause liver damage.

VITAMINS Vitamins are best when they come from a varied, healthful diet. Headache sufferers who would like to improve their vitamin status should ask their doctor about supplements. The most commonly recommended supplement for headaches is vitamin B_6, 50 or 100 mg per day. Some people claim they can help ward off an oncoming headache with 50 mg of niacin, though this can cause headaches in others. Although vitamin E has been used for headaches, it probably does not have much impact. Low magnesium levels may be linked to menstrual migraines; important dietary sources include nuts, legumes, and dark green vegetables.

HOMEOPATHIC REMEDIES

Homeopathic reference books list a handful of remedies based on the source of a headache, such as a missed meal or eyestrain. While homeopathic medications are *usually* safe, some cases have linked them to liver or muscle problems.

Unfortunately, few well-conducted, large, and controlled studies have assessed the effectiveness of the various remedies because such testing is very costly. Although some anecdotes about therapies sound promising, without controlled studies, we cannot draw conclusions.

Some of these natural medications have a place in the treatment of headaches, but which ones will ultimately prove most effective is still unclear. We compiled the following recommendations from several different sources. Many of these substances are available at health food stores or homeopathic pharmacies.

- Migraines: *Feverfew leaves* (one of the most widely used natural remedies); *garlic* and *ginger* pills
- Headaches from colds, noise, or light; pain in the temples or the entire right half of head; any headache with intense, throbbing pain: *Belladonna 9C (the concentration)*
- Menopausal headaches: *Lachesis 9C*
- Headaches related to periods (before, during, or after): *Natrum muriaticum* or *Pulsatilla*
- Headaches accompanied by visual disturbances, nausea, or vomiting: *Iris versicolor 9C, Natrum muriaticum, Phosphorus, Tuberculinum,* or *Sulphur*
- Headaches accompanied by dizziness and a weakening of sight: *Kali phosphoricum*
- Headaches accompanied with dizziness and blurred vision: *Magnesia phosphorica*
- Headaches that start at the back of the head and occur after visual disturbances, with pain settling on right side: *Gelsemium* or *Sanguinaria*
- Headaches after a head injury: *Natrum sulphuricum*

- Headaches with diarrhea or cold sweats: *Veratrum album* 9C
- Chronic tension headaches: *Tuberculinum*
- Headaches that are aggravated by moving the head or eyes, usually characterized by a steady ache (rather than throbbing): *Bryonia*
- Headaches triggered by alcohol (including hangover headaches), coffee, or other drugs; by overeating or undersleeping, excessive concentration, or mental strain: *Nux vomica*

MASSAGE AND STRETCHES

Massage to the neck and lower skull area benefits many headache sufferers by easing painful knots, but the benefits are usually short-lived. Full-body or face massages may help by relaxing you, whereas massaging the forehead, temple, back of the neck, and shoulders may be particularly useful for tension headaches.

You can also relax these areas with some stretching exercises that involve the neck (rolling your head, gently pressing it forward with your hands at the base of your skull, rolling and shrugging your shoulders).

SEX

Believe it or not, sexual intercourse was found to help relieve migraines in about half the women studied in a research project at the Southern Illinois University School of Medicine. Men were not evaluated in the study, but for some the release of tension from intercourse just may help.

HEADBANDS

When migraine sufferers get some relief by pressing the side of the head near the pain, another simple measure might help: wearing any snug elastic band around the head. According to an article in *American Family Physician* (vol. 47, no. 1, 1993, p. 11), these headbands helped about one-quarter of the study participants, who obtained at least 50 percent relief.

IMPROVING POSTURE

Positions that strain the neck, such as sitting at a computer for long periods, may contribute to headache pain. Adjust the seat and table so your neck is not bent or extended. Take breaks every fifteen minutes or so; do two minutes of stretching every two or three hours. Regular stretching of the neck and lower back can decrease headaches.

THE HEADACHE FRONTIER

Most medications now used for headaches were developed for other purposes and then accidentally discovered to help headaches too. Chances are, some headache drugs of the future will be medications already on the market for other purposes.

In development, however, are new drugs that focus primarily on the serotonin system in the brain. One promising medication that may prevent migraines is sergolexole maleate, now being tested by Eli Lilly and Company. It appears to prevent blood vessel dilation through a serotonin mechanism.

The immune system may also be a fertile ground for new drug strategies. Scientists have uncovered evidence that a significant number of headache patients have lower numbers of immune cells called suppressors, implying an overactive immune system. Unrelated to allergies that are linked to the immune system, these cells counter the actions of helper cells in the immune response. Although certain drugs, such as the corticosteroids Prednisone, Decadron, and Depo-Medrol, help migraine and cluster headaches for a brief time via the immune system, they have a wide array of side effects and their benefits tend to wane if used for long periods. The challenge is to develop safe but effective medications that alter the immune system in a way that helps headache patients and are deemed safe for long-term use.

As researchers get closer to discovering the gene that is responsible for inherited headaches, it may someday even be possible to alter genes to decrease migraine and tension headaches. Of course, scientists and patients must address many ethical and moral questions before undertaking gene therapy.

In the next thirty years, we will probably see more and more studies assessing the benefits of alternative treatments, such as homeopathic remedies, sorting out which treatments are effective and worthwhile.

PUTTING IT ALL TOGETHER

This book is chock full of advice and information that your doctor may consider for your headaches. We cannot stress strongly enough, however, that your own management techniques can go a very long way toward reducing the frequency and severity of headaches. To recap, we want to leave you with these final suggestions:

- Learn how to cope with stress effectively, whether through cognitive strategies that can be learned from self-help books or in a few sessions of psychotherapy, relaxation and breathing techniques, exercise, yoga, massage, footbaths, or whatever works for you. Don't overload yourself with too many obligations. Learn to say no.
- Exercise regularly. Aerobic exercise — as little as twenty minutes of brisk walking three or four times a week — and daily neck and back stretches can help ward off headaches.
- Pay attention to your diet. Keep track and limit foods that trigger your headaches. Eat regularly and healthfully (plenty of whole

grains, pasta, fruits and vegetables; limit sugar, salt, and fat), do not skip meals, and drink a lot of water.

- Maintain a regular sleeping schedule. Try to wake up at the same time every day; sleeping late may trigger a headache.
- Avoid or limit alcohol, especially types that you know can trigger headaches.
- Control environmental factors that may trigger your headaches: avoid smoky rooms, fumes, and perfumes, for instance.
- See a doctor if you get headaches that interfere with your life.

APPENDICES

REFERENCES

INDEX

•

APPENDIX A:
HEADACHE
ASSOCIATIONS

· · · · · · · ·

∼∼∼∼

The following associations and foundations offer free or inexpensive materials on headaches.

FOR HEADACHE INFORMATION AND REFERRALS

The National Headache Foundation
5252 North Western Avenue, Department PF
Chicago, Illinois 60625
312-878-7715 or 800-843-2256

By sending a self-addressed envelope stamped with 55 cents postage, you may request a copy of the brochure "Plain Facts About Migraines: Symptoms and Treatments." For small fees, the NHF also offers several brochures and booklets, as well as relaxation audiotapes.

For $15 a year, you will receive a quarterly newsletter on the late developments in headache research and treatment.

The American Council for Headache Education (ACHE)
875 Kings Highway
West Deptford, New Jersey 08096
800-255-ACHE

By calling the toll-free number, you can obtain general information, help in starting a local headache support group, and referrals to doctors who take a special interest in headaches and belong to the American Association for the Study of Headache (AASH). For $15 a year, you can subscribe to a quarterly newsletter on the latest developments in the headache field.

TO START A HEADACHE SUPPORT GROUP

Sharing experiences and tips with others who face similar challenges can help you cope. Once you realize that you are far from alone in dealing with headache problems, you will feel more in control over your life and confident about your decisions.

ACHE and NHF can both help. So can the following organization, which locates local self-help groups.

National Self-Help Clearinghouse
25 West 43d Street
New York, New York 10036
212-354-8525

Another organization can help you find specific medical programs in your area.

American Self-Help Clearinghouse
St. Clares–Riverside Medical Center
25 Pocono Road
Denville, New Jersey 07834
201-625-7101

TO DO MORE RESEARCH

To understand headache medication better, consider checking current reference books in the library (where you'll probably have access to a photocopy machine) or at your pharmacist's office. The *Physicians' Desk Reference* is just one of several guides to prescription medications. You can also check a doctor's credentials through a directory of physicians or medical specialists.

If you want to know about recently published studies regarding headache research, you can access medical databases through a public library or medical library. Ask the librarian to help you access Medline (a specific database) or MEDLARS (an umbrella database comprised of about forty specific databases). Usually for a fee, reference librarians will design and conduct a search for you. You need to be cautious in reading medical studies, however; the papers are highly technical and sometimes based on poorly conducted studies. Also, the conclusions of isolated studies often need to be put into perspective. It is difficult for the lay reader to generalize one study's results to treatment without previous knowledge about other publications in the field. Nevertheless, becoming familiar with the research can help consumers question their doctors more aggressively.

All these searches will result in a bibliography with citations and abstracts of journal articles on specific topics published in the medical literature.

HELP BY PHONE

To access medically oriented tape-recorded messages on medical topics, including relaxation and stress management, call or write:

TEL-MED The Health Line
952 South Mount Vernon Avenue
Colton, California 92324
714-825-6034

MIND-BODY APPROACHES

We cannot stress enough the importance of relaxation and coping exercises in relieving and preventing headaches. For more information on these topics, consider the public library, which probably has many tapes and books on relaxation, stress reduction, coping strategies, deep-breathing exercises, and so on, or contact one of the following organizations.

HYPNOSIS

American Society for Clinical Hypnosis
2200 East Devon Avenue, Suite 291
Des Plaines, Illinois 60018
708-297-3317

Society for Clinical and Experimental Hypnosis
129A King's Park Drive
Liverpool, New York 13090
315-652-7299

This organization has a membership of 1,100 professionals.

The American Council of Hypnotist Examiners
1147 East Broadway, Suite 340
Glendale, California 91205
818-242-5378

ACUPUNCTURE
To obtain referrals close to your area, contact:

American Academy of Medical Acupuncture
58200 Wilshire Boulevard, Suite 500
Los Angeles, California 90036
213-937-5514

American Association of Acupuncture and Oriental
Medicine
1400 16th Street, N.W., Suite 710
Washington, D.C. 20036
202-265-2276

BIOFEEDBACK
To obtain information and referrals, contact:

Association for Applied Psychophysiology and Feedback
(formerly The Biofeedback Society of America) and
The Biofeedback Certification Institute of America
10200 West 44th Avenue, Suite 304
Wheatridge, Colorado 80033
303-422-8436 (AAPF)
303-420-2902 (BCIA)

MINDFULNESS-BASED STRESS REDUCTION
Audiotapes on this technique are available from:

Stress Reduction Tapes
P.O. Box 547
Lexington, Massachusetts 02173

For information about five-day and eight-week training sessions, contact:

The Stress Reduction Clinic at the University of Massachusetts Medical Center
55 Lake Avenue North
Worcester, Massachusetts 01655
508-856-1616

GENERAL MIND-BODY INFORMATION

For general information on mind-body research, contact:

The Fetzer Institute
9292 West KL Avenue
Kalamazoo, Michigan 49009
616-375-2000

Center for Mind-Body Medicine
5225 Connecticut Avenue, N.W., Suite 414
Washington, D.C. 20015
202-966-7338

HERBAL MEDICINE

American Botanical Council
P.O. Box 201660
Austin, Texas 78720
Fax: 512-331-1924

CHINESE MEDICINE

American Foundation of Traditional Chinese Medicine
505 Beach Street
San Francisco, California 94133
415-776-0502

COUNSELING AND PSYCHOTHERAPY

To find a therapy referral, ask your doctor for the name of a psychiatrist, clinical psychologist, or psychiatric social worker. National organizations that might have local branches or can offer referrals include:

American Psychiatric Association
1400 K Street, N.W.
Washington, D.C. 20005
202-682-6000

American Psychological Association
750 First Street, N.E.
Washington, D.C. 20002
202-336-5700

National Association of Social Workers
750 First Street, N.E., Suite 700
Washington, D.C. 20002
202-408-8600

Center for Cognitive Therapy
Science Center, Room 754
3600 Market Street
Philadelphia, Pennsylvania 19104
215-898-4100

APPENDIX B:
OVER-THE-COUNTER
HEADACHE MEDICATIONS

• • • • • • • •

~~~~~

The following table lists the most common over-the-counter headache medications and their composition. You may compare medications, for example, by their caffeine content and whether they contain acetaminophen or aspirin. By knowing how much of a compound these medications contain, you can compare their relative strength and their likelihood of giving you discomfort if you are sensitive, for example, to aspirin.

Note: Pseudoephedrine is a vasocontrictor (blood vessel constrictor) of the upper respiratory tract; as a result, it helps shrink swollen tissues in the sinuses and nose.

OVER-THE-COUNTER HEADACHE MEDICATIONS

Brand-name Medication	Aspirin	Aceta-minophen	Ibuprofen	Caffeine	Pseudo-ephedrine	Other
Aspirin Free Anacin Caplets		500 mg				
Aspirin Free Anacin Tablets		500 mg				
Aspirin Free Anacin P.M. Caplets		500 mg				diphenhydramine hydrochloride 25 mg
Bayer Select Headache Pain Relief		500 mg		65 mg		
Bayer Select Menstrual Multi-Symptom Formula		500 mg				parabrom 25 mg
Bayer Select Night Time Pain Relief		500 mg				diphenhydramine hydrochloride 25 mg
Bufferin AF Nite Time Analgesic/Sleeping Aid Caplets		500 mg				diphenhydramine citrate 38 mg
Aspirin Free Excedrin Analgesic Caplets		500 mg		65 mg		
Excedrin Extra-Strength Analgesic Tablets and Caplets	250 mg	250 mg		65 mg		
Excedrin P.M. Analgesic/Sleeping Aid		500 mg				diphenhydramine citrate 38 mg
Maximum Strength Multi-Symptom Menstrual Formula Midol		500 mg		60 mg		pyrilamine maleate 15 mg
PMS Multi-Symptom Formula Midol		500 mg				parabrom 25 mg pyrilamine maleate 15 mg
Regular Strength Multi-Symptom Midol Formula		325 mg				pyrilamine maleate 15 mg
Multi-Symptom Pamprin Tablets and Caplets		500 mg				parabrom 25 mg pyrilamine maleate 15 mg

OVER-THE-COUNTER HEADACHE MEDICATIONS

Brand-name Medication	Aspirin	Aceta-minophen	Ibuprofen	Caffeine	Pseudo-ephedrine	Other
Maximum Pain Relief Pamprin Caplets		250 mg				magnesium salicylate 250 mg, parabrom 25 mg
Maximum Strength Panadol Tablets and Caplets		500 mg				
Percogesic Analgesic Tablets		325 mg				phenyltoloxamine citrate 30 mg
Sominex Pain Relief Formula		500 mg				diphenhydramine hydrochloride 25 mg
St. Joseph Aspirin-Free Fever Reducer for Children Chewable Tablets		80 mg				
Tylenol Children's Chewable Tablets, Elixir, and Suspension Liquid		Tablets 80 mg Elixir 160 mg (5 ml) Liquid 160 mg (5 ml)				
Tylenol Extra Strength, Adult Liquid Pain Reliever		15 ml–500 mg				
Tylenol Extra Strength, Gelcaps, Caplets, and Tablets		500 mg				
Tylenol Headache Plus Pain Reliever and Antacid Caplets		500 mg				calcium carbonate 250 mg
Tylenol Junior Strength, Coated Caplets, Grape and Fruit Chewable Tablets		160 mg				
Tylenol Regular Strength, Caplets and Tablets		325 mg				

OVER-THE-COUNTER HEADACHE MEDICATIONS

Brand-name Medication	Aspirin	Aceta-minophen	Ibuprofen	Caffeine	Pseudo-ephedrine	Other
Tylenol PM Extra Strength Pain Reliever/ Sleep Aid Gelcaps, Caplets, and Tablets		500 mg				diphenhydramine hydrochloride 25 mg
Unisom with Pain Relief Nighttime Sleep Aid/Analgesic		650 mg				diphenhydramine hydrochloride 50 mg
Vanquish Analgesic Caplets	227 mg	194 mg		33 mg		dried aluminum hydroxide gel 25 mg, magnesium hydroxide 50 mg
Tylenol Headache Plus Pain Reliever with Antacid Caplets		500 mg				calcium carbonate 250 mg
Bayer Children's Chewable Aspirin	81 mg					
Genuine Bayer Aspirin Tablets and Caplets	325 mg					hydroxypropyl methylcellulose coating for easier swallowing
Maximum Bayer Aspirin Tablets and Caplets	500 mg					hydroxypropyl methylcellulose coating for easier swallowing
Extended Release Bayer 8-Hour Aspirin	650 mg					
Adult Low Strength Enteric Aspirin Tablets	81 mg					
Regular Strength Bayer Enteric Aspirin Caplets	325 mg					
Empirin Aspirin	325 mg					
Norwich Aspirin	325 mg					
Norwich Aspirin Maximum Strength	500 mg					

OVER-THE-COUNTER HEADACHE MEDICATIONS

Brand-name Medication	Aspirin	Aceta-minophen	Ibuprofen	Caffeine	Pseudo-ephedrine	Other
Norwich Enteric Safety Coated Aspirin	325 mg					
Norwich Enteric Safety Coated Aspirin Maximum Strength	500 mg					
St. Joseph Adult Chewable Aspirin	81 mg					
Anacin Caplets	400 mg			32 mg		
Anacin Tablets	400 mg			32 mg		
Maximum Strength Anacin Tablets	500 mg			32 mg		
Arthritis Strength BC Powder	742 mg			36 mg		salicylamide 222 mg
Ascriptin A/D Caplets	325 mg					buffered with Maalox (alumina-magnesia) and calcium carbonate
Extra Strength Ascriptin Caplets	500 mg					buffered with Maalox (alumina-magnesia) and calcium carbonate
Regular Strength Ascriptin Tablets	325 mg					buffered with Maalox (alumina-magnesia) and calcium carbonate
BC Powder	650 mg			32 mg		salicylamide 195 mg
BC Cold Powder Multi-Symptom Formula (Cold-Sinus-Allergy)	650 mg					phenylpropano-lamine hydrochloride 25 mg, chlorphenira-mine maleate 4 mg
BC Cold Powder Non-Drowsy Formula (Cold-Sinus)	650 mg					phenylpropano-lamine hydrochlo-ride 25 mg

OVER-THE-COUNTER HEADACHE MEDICATIONS

Brand-name Medication	Aspirin	Aceta- minophen	Ibuprofen	Caffeine	Pseudo- ephedrine	Other
Bayer Plus Aspirin Tablets	325 mg					buffered with calcium carbonate, magnesium carbonate, magnesium oxide
Extra Strength Bayer Plus Aspirin Caplets	500 mg					buffered with calcium carbonate, magnesium carbonate, magnesium oxide
Arthritis Strength Bufferin Analgesic Caplets	500 mg					buffered with calcium carbonate, magnesium carbonate, magnesium oxide
Extra Strength Bufferin Analgesic Tablets	500 mg					buffered with calcium carbonate, magnesium carbonate, magnesium oxide
Bufferin Analgesic Tablets and Caplets	325 mg					buffered with calcium carbonate, magnesium carbonate, magnesium oxide
Cama Arthritis Pain Reliever	500 mg					magnesium oxide 150 mg, aluminum hydroxide 125 mg
Ecotrin Enteric Coated Aspirin Maximum Strength Tablets and Caplets	500 mg					acetylsalicylic acid
Ecotrin Enteric Coated Aspirin Regular Strength Tablets and Caplets	325 mg					acetylsalicylic acid
Excedrin Extra- Strength Analgesic Tablets and Caplets	250 mg	250 mg		65 mg		

OVER-THE-COUNTER HEADACHE MEDICATIONS

Brand-name Medication	Aspirin	Aceta-minophen	Ibuprofen	Caffeine	Pseudo-ephedrine	Other
P-A-C Analgesic Tablets	400 mg			caffeine anhy-drous 32 mg		
Ursinus Inlay-Tabs	325 mg				30 mg	
Vanquish Analgesic Caplets	227 mg	194 mg		33 mg		dried aluminum hy-droxide gel 25 mg, magnesium hydrox-ide 50 mg
Aleve Tablets						naproxen 220 mg
Alka-Seltzer Efferve-scent Antacid and Pain Reliever	325 mg					heat-treated sodium bicarbonate 1916 mg, citric acid 1000 mg
Alka-Seltzer Extra Strength Efferves-cent Antacid and Pain Reliever	500 mg					heat-treated sodium bicarbonate 1985 mg, citric acid 1000 mg
Alka-Seltzer (Flavored) Effervescent Antacid and Pain Reliever	325 mg					heat-treated sodium bicarbonate 1710 mg, citric acid 1220 mg
Regular Strength Ascriptin Tablets	325 mg					buffered with Maalox (alumina-magnesia) and cal-cium carbonate
Advil Ibuprofen Caplets and Tablets			200 mg			
Bayer Select Ibu-profen Pain Relief Formula			200 mg			
Haltran Tablets			200 mg			
Ibuprohm Ibuprofen Caplets			200 mg			
Ibuprohm Ibuprofen Tablets			200 mg			

OVER-THE-COUNTER HEADACHE MEDICATIONS

Brand-name Medication	Aspirin	Aceta-minophen	Ibuprofen	Caffeine	Pseudo-ephedrine	Other
Motrin IB Caplets and Tablets			200 mg			
Nuprin Ibuprofen/ Analgesic Tablets and Caplets			200 mg			
Extra Strength Doan's P.M.						magnesium salicylate 500 mg, diphenhydramine hydrochloride 25 mg
Mobigesic Analgesic Tablets						magnesium salicylate 325 mg, phenyltoloxamine citrate 30 mg
Actifed Plus Caplets		500 mg			30 mg	triprolidine hydrochloride 1.25 mg
Actifed Plus Tablets		500 mg			30 mg	triprolidine hydrochloride 1.25 mg
Actifed Sinus Daytime/Nighttime Caplets		Daytime 325 mg, Nighttime 500 mg			Daytime 30 mg, Nighttime 30 mg	diphenhydramine hydrochloride 25 mg
Actifed Sinus Daytime/Nighttime Tablets		Daytime 325 mg, Nighttime 500 mg			Daytime 30 mg, Nighttime 30 mg	diphenhydramine hydrochloride 25 mg
Advil Cold and Sinus (formerly CoAdvil)			200 mg		30 mg	
Bayer Select Sinus Pain Relief Formula		500 mg			30 mg	
Chlor-Trimeton Allergy-Sinus Headache Caplets		500 mg				chlorpheniramine maleate 2 mg, phenylpropanolamine hydrochloride, 12.5 mg

OVER-THE-COUNTER HEADACHE MEDICATIONS

Brand-name Medication	Aspirin	Aceta-minophen	Ibuprofen	Caffeine	Pseudo-ephedrine	Other
Comtrex Multi-Symptom Cold Reliever Tablets, Caplets, Liqui-Gels, and Liquid		Tablet 325 mg, Caplet 325 mg Liqui-gel 325 mg Liquid 650 mg			Tablet 30 mg, Caplet 30 mg Liquid 60 mg	phenylpropanol-amine hydrochloride (Liqui-gel only) 12.5 mg chlorpheniramine maleate (Tablet, Caplet, and Liqui-gel 2 mg, Liquid 4 mg) dextromethorphan (Tablet, Caplet, and Liqui-gel 10 mg, Liquid 20 mg)
Comtrex Multi-Symptom Non-Drowsy Caplets		325 mg			30 mg	dextromethorphan hydrobromide 10 mg
Dimetapp Sinus Caplets			200 mg		30 mg	
Dristan Sinus			200 mg		30 mg	
Sinus Excedrin Analgesic Decon-gestant Tablets and Caplets		500 mg			30 mg	
Sinarest No Drowsiness Tablets		500 mg			30 mg	
Sinarest Tablets		325 mg			30 mg	chlorpheniramine maleate 2 mg
Sinarest Extra Strength Tablets		500 mg			30 mg	chlorpheniramine maleate 2 mg
Sine-Aid Maxi-mum Strength Sinus Headache Gelcaps, Caplets, and Tablets		500 mg			30 mg	

OVER-THE-COUNTER HEADACHE MEDICATIONS

Brand-name Medication	Aspirin	Aceta-minophen	Ibuprofen	Caffeine	Pseudo-ephedrine	Other
Sine-Off Maximum Strength No Drowsiness Formula Caplets			500 mg		30 mg	
Sine-Off Sinus Medicine Tablets Aspirin Formula	325 mg					chlorpheniramine maleate 2 mg phenylpropanol-amine hydrochloride 12.5 mg
Sinutab Sinus Allergy Medication, Maximum Strength Caplets		500 mg			30 mg	chlorpheniramine maleate 2 mg
Sinutab Sinus Medication, Maximum Strength without Drowsiness Formula, Tablets and Caplets		500 mg			30 mg	
Sinutab Sinus Medication, Regular Strength without Drowsiness Formula		325 mg			30 mg	
Sudafed Plus Tablets					60 mg	chlorpheniramine maleate 4 mg
Sudafed Sinus Caplets		500 mg			30 mg	
Tylenol Allergy Sinus Medication Maximum Strength Gelcaps and Caplets		500 mg			30 mg	chlorpheniramine maleate 2 mg
Tylenol Cold Medication No Drowsiness Formula Gelcaps and Caplets		325 mg			30 mg	dextromethorphan hydrobromide 15 mg
Tylenol Cold Night Time Medication		650 mg/ 30 ml			60 mg/ 30 ml	diphenhydramine hydrochloride 50 mg/30 ml

OVER-THE-COUNTER HEADACHE MEDICATIONS

Brand-name Medication	Aspirin	Aceta- minophen	Ibuprofen	Caffeine	Pseudo- ephedrine	Other
Tylenol, Maximum Strength, Sinus Medication Gelcaps, Caplets, and Tablets		500 mg			30 mg	
Benadryl Allergy Sinus Headache Formula		500 mg			30 mg	diphenhydramine hydrochloride 12.5 mg
Allergy-Sinus Comtrex Multi-Symptom Allergy-Sinus Formula Tablets and Caplets		500 mg			30 mg	chlorpheniramine maleate 2 mg
Sinus Excedrin Analgesic, Decongestant Tablets and Caplets		500 mg			30 mg	
BRAND-NAME ANTINAUSEA MEDICATION						
Dramamine Chewable Tablets						dimenhydrinate 50 mg
Dramamine Tablets						dimenhydrinate 50 mg
Emetrol						5 ml teaspoonful: dextrose 1.87 g, levulose 1.87 g, phosphor acid 21.5 mg
Marezine Tablets						cyclizine hydrochloride 50 mg
Pepto-Bismol Liquid						15 ml: bismuth subsalicylate 262 mg, salicylate 130 mg
Pepto-Bismol Tablets						bismuth subsalicylate 262 mg, salicylate 102 mg

APPENDIX C: PRESCRIPTION
HEADACHE MEDICATIONS

• • • • • • • •

For your reference, here is a list of prescription analgesics and sedatives for headache and their composition. In some cases we have listed the milligram content of ingredients for easy comparison to similar medications.

BRAND NAME	COMPOSITION
Anexsia 5/500	hydrocodone bitartrate 5 mg, acetaminophen 500 mg
Anexsia 7.5/650	hydrocodone bitartrate 7.5 mg, acetaminophen 650 mg
Ativan	lorazepam
Axotal	butalbital 50 mg, aspirin 650 mg
B-A-C	butalbital 50 mg, aspirin 650 mg caffeine 40 mg
Bancap HC	hydrocodone bitartrate 5 mg, acetaminophen 500 mg
Centrax	prazepam
Co-Gesic	hydrocodone bitartrate 5 mg, acetaminophen 500 mg
Damason-P	hydrocodone bitartrate 5 mg, aspirin 224 mg, caffeine 32 mg
Darvocet-N 100	propoxyphene napsylate 100 mg, acetaminophen 650 mg

BRAND NAME	COMPOSITION
Darvon Compound	propoxyphene hydrochloride 32 mg, aspirin 389 mg, caffeine 32.4 mg
Darvon Compound-65	propoxyphene hydrochloride 65 mg, aspirin 389 mg, caffeine 43.4 mg
Demerol	meperidine hydrochloride
Dilaudid	hydromorphone hydrochloride
Dolophine Hydrochloride	methadone hydrochloride
DuoCet	hydrocodone bitartrate 5 mg, acetaminophen 500 mg
Empirin with Codeine 2	codeine 15 mg, aspirin 325 mg
Empirin with Codeine 3	codeine 30 mg, aspirin 325 mg
Empirin with Codeine 4	codeine 60 mg, aspirin 325 mg
Esgic	butalbital 50 mg, acetaminophen 325 mg, caffeine 40 mg
Fioricet	butalbital 50 mg, acetaminophen 325 mg, caffeine 40 mg
Fioricet with codeine	butalbital 50 mg, acetaminophen 325 mg, caffeine 40 mg, codeine 30 mg
Fiorinal	butalbital 50 mg, aspirin 325 mg, caffeine 40 mg
Fiorinal with Codeine 3	butalbital 50 mg, aspirin 325 mg, caffeine 40 mg, codeine 30 mg
Hydrocet	hydrocodone bitartrate 5 mg, acetaminophen 500 mg
Klonopin	clonazepam

BRAND NAME	COMPOSITION
Levo-Dromoran	levorphanol tartrate
Librium	chlordiazepoxide
Mepergan	meperidine hydrochloride, promethazine hydrochloride
Nubain	nalbuphine hydrochloride
Percocet	oxycodone 5 mg, acetaminophen 325 mg
Percodan	oxycodone hydrochloride 4.5 mg, oxycodone terephthalate 0.38 mg, aspirin 325 mg
Phenaphen 2	acetaminophen 325 mg, codeine 15 mg
Phenaphen 3	acetaminophen 325 mg, codeine 30 mg
Phenaphen 4	acetaminophen 325 mg, codeine 60 mg
Phenobarbital	phenobarbital
Phrenilin	butalbital 50 mg, acetaminophen 325 mg
Phrenilin Forte	butalbital 50 mg, acetaminophen 650 mg
Serax	oxazepam
Stadol	butorphanol tartrate
Synalgos-DC	dihydrocodeine bitartrate 16 mg, aspirin 356.4 mg, caffeine 30 mg
Talacen	pentazocine hydrochloride 25 mg, acetaminophen 650 mg
Talwin Compound	pentazocine hydrochloride 12.5 mg, aspirin 325 mg
Talwin Nx	pentazocine hydrochloride 50 mg, naloxone hydrochloride 0.5 mg
Tranxene	clorazepate

BRAND NAME	COMPOSITION
Tylenol 2	acetaminophen 300 mg, codeine 15 mg
Tylenol 3	acetaminophen 300 mg, codeine 30 mg
Tylenol 4	acetaminophen 300 mg, codeine 60 mg
Tylox	oxycodone 5 mg, acetaminophen 500 mg
Valium	diazepam
Valrelease	diazepam
Vicodin	hydrocodone bitartrate 5 mg, acetaminophen 500 mg
Wygesic	propoxyphene hydrochloride 65 mg, acetaminophen 650 mg
Xanax	alprazolam
Zydone	hydrocodone bitartrate 5 mg, acetaminophen 500 mg

REFERENCES

· · · · · · · · ·

FOR THE TECHNICAL READER

BOOKS
Bourne, Edmond J., Ph.D. *The Anxiety and Phobia Workbook.* Oakland, Calif.: New Harbinger Publications, 1990.

Diamond, Seymour, and Donald J. Dalessio. *The Practicing Physician's Approach to Headache.* 5th ed. Baltimore: Williams and Wilkins, 1992.

Raskin, Neil. *Headache.* 2d ed. New York: Churchill Livingstone, 1988.

Robbins, Lawrence D., M.D. *Management of Headache and Headache Medication.* New York: Springer-Verlag, 1993.

Sheehan, David. *The Anxiety Disease.* New York: Bantam Books, 1983.

ARTICLES
Brew, B. J, and J. Miller. "New Trouble for AIDS Patients: Severe Headache with No Cause." *Consultant* (December 1993): 92.

Cady, Roger K., and C. Normal Shealy. "Recent Advances in Migraine Management." *Journal of Family Practice,* vol. 36 (January 1993): 85–92.

Derman, Howard S., "Migraine Headaches: How to Track Diagnostic Clues and Tailor Therapy." *Consultant* (June 1993): 113–22.

"Headache and Depression (Tips from Other Journals)." *American Family Physician,* vol. 43 (February 1991): 660.

Hering, R., and T. J. Steiner. "Abrupt Outpatient Withdrawal of Medication in Analgesic-Abusing Migraineurs." *The Lancet,* vol. 337 (15 June 1991): 1442–43.

Ostergaard, John R., and Morten Kraft. "Natural Course of Benign Coital Headache." *British Medical Journal,* vol. 305 (7 November 1992): 1129.

Purath, Janet. "Assessing Headache Pain." *RN,* vol. 54 (October 1991): 26–32.

Robbins, Lawrence, M.D. "Precipitating Factors in Migraines: A Retrospective Review of 494 Patients." *Headache,* vol. 34 (April 1994): 214–16.

Trachtenbarg, David E., and Cris J. Presutti. "Uncovering Clues That Suggest a Malevolent Cause (Headaches)." *Consultant* (September 1993): 146–50.

FOR THE GENERAL READER

BOOKS

American Council For Headache Education (ACHE), with Lynne Constantine and Suzanne Scott. *Migraine: The Complete Guide.* New York: Dell, 1994.

Anderson, Bob. *Stretching.* Bolinas, Calif.: Shelter, 1980.

Benson, Herbert, M.D. *The Relaxation Response.* New York: Morrow, 1975.

Lipton, Richard B., M.D., Lawrence C. Newman, M.D., and Helene MacLean. *Migraine: Beating the Odds. The Doctors' Guide to Reducing Your Risk.* Reading, Mass.: Addison-Wesley, 1992.

Rapoport, Alan M., M.D., and Fred D. Sheftell, M.D. *Headache Relief.* New York: Fireside, 1990.

Sacks, Oliver, M.D. *Migraine: Understanding a Common Disorder.* Berkeley, Calif.: University of California Press, 1985.

Saper, Joel R., and Kenneth R. Magee. *Freedom from Headaches: A Personal Guide for Understanding and Treating Headache, Face and Neck Pain.* New York: Simon and Schuster, 1978.

Solomon, Seymour, M.D., and Steven Fraccaro. *The Headache Book.* Yonkers, N.Y.: Consumer Reports Books, 1991.

ON HOMEOPATHIC MEDICINE

Coulter, Catherine. *Portraits of Homeopathic Medicines,* vol. 2. Berkeley, Calif.: North Atlantic Books, 1988.

Cummings, Stephen, and Dana Ullman. *Everybody's Guide to Homeopathic Medicine.* Los Angeles: Jeremy Tarcher, 1984.

Herscu, Paul, M.D. *The Homeopathic Treatment of Children.* Berkeley, Calif.: North Atlantic Books, 1991.

Horvilleur, Alain, M.D. *The Family Guide to Homeopathy.* Norwood, Pa.: Health and Homeopathy Publishing, 1986.

Monte, Tom. "30 Powerful Natural Remedies." *Natural Health,* vol. 23 (May–June 1993): 78–82.

Natra-Bio Homeopathic Reference Manual. Ferndale, Wash.

ACKNOWLEDGMENTS

· · · · · · · ·

I would like to first thank my coauthor, Susan, and our editor, Gail. I want to thank my dad, Joseph, for continuing support. I want to thank my children, Mark, Michelle, and Michael, and their mom, Sharon. And finally, thank you to my wonderful staff at the Robbins Headache Clinic for their continuing hard work and support, particularly Dorrie, Barb, Karen, and Phyllis.

— L.D.R.

First I want to thank Larry Bernard of the Cornell News Service for connecting me with my coauthor. I want to thank Bob Silverstein, my agent, for finding a publisher; Gail Winston, our editor, for believing in the project; and Jayne Yaffe, our manuscript editor, for her meticulous attention to detail and help in shaping the book. I want to thank my dad, Solon J. Lang, for his love, intellectual guidance, and support over the years. And I want to thank my husband, Tom Schneider, and my daughter, Julia Lang Schneider, for their continuing love and support.

— S.S.L.

INDEX

· · · · · ·

Abortive medications, 9; addiction to, 9; for adolescents' headaches, 179–82; for children's headaches, 167–76; for cluster headaches, 148–52; development of, 212–13; for migraines, 59, 62–74; for post-traumatic headaches, 191; side effects of, 9; for tension headaches, 124–27

Accidents. *See* Post-traumatic headaches

Acetaminophen: for adolescents' headaches, 180; for after-surgery headaches, 199; in Anacin, 30; for children's headaches, 168–69; description of, 33; in Excedrin Extra-Strength, 30, 181; in Midrin, 64, 126, 171; in over-the-counter pain relievers, 30; during pregnancy, 227; and rebound headaches, 8, 124; as a self-help strategy, 19; for tension headaches, 124

Acetaminophen with codeine, 72, 117, 237, 238. *See also* Narcotics

Acetaminophen with hydrocodone, 73

ACTH (adrenocorticotropic hormone), 72, 153. *See also* Corticosteroids; Cortisone

Actifed Plus, 231

Actifed Sinus Daytime/Nighttime, 231

Acupressure, 207–8

Acupuncture, 206–7, 221

Addiction: to abortive medications, 9, 126, 150; to amphetamines, 136; to butalbital compounds, 181; to cocaine,

157; to muscle relaxants, 133; to tranquilizers, 136. *See also* Narcotics

Adolescents' headaches. *See* Children's headaches

Adrenocorticotropic hormone (ACTH), 72, 153. *See also* Corticosteroids; Cortisone

Advil: for children's headaches, 169; composition of, 231; description of, 31–32, 230; in liquid form, 169; for migraines, 64; and rebound headaches, 8; as a self-help strategy, 19; for tension headaches, 125, 132. *See also* Ibuprofen

Aerobic exercise, 22, 213

After-surgery headaches, 199

Alcohol, 7, 86, 112, 147, 196, 200, 211, 214

Aleve: for adolescents' headaches, 180; for children's headaches, 171; description of, 31, 230; for migraines, 99–100; for tension headaches, 125, 132. *See also* Naproxen

Alka-Seltzer, 230

Allergy headaches, 12, 15, 196

Alprazolam, 238

Alternative headache remedies, 205–14

Altitude, 72, 83, 90

American Academy of Medical Acupuncture, 207, 221

American Association for the Study of Headache (AASH), 218

American Association of Acupuncture and Oriental Medicine, 221

American Botanical Council, 222
American Council for Headache Education (ACHE), 217–18
American Council of Hypnotist Examiners, 220
American Foundation of Traditional Chinese Medicine, 222
American Psychiatric Association, 222
American Psychological Association, 222
American Self-Help Clearinghouse, 218
American Society for Clinical Hypnosis, 220
Amines, 85
Amitriptyline: for adolescents' headaches, 182–83; for children's headaches, 178–79; headaches caused by, 202; for hemicrania continua, 200; for migraines, 92–93, 102, 118; for posttraumatic headaches, 192; for tension headaches, 130. *See also* Antidepressants
Amitriptyline with propranolol, 102, 135
Amphetamines, 136
Anacin, 29, 30, 33, 180, 228
Anacin Maximum-Strength, 33, 228
Analgesics. *See* Acetaminophen; Aspirin
Anaprox: for adolescents' headaches, 180; for children's headaches, 171; description of, 31; for exercise headaches, 193; for migraines, 99–100; for tension headaches, 132. *See also* Naproxen
Anaprox DS, 63–64, 125, 150. *See also* Naproxen
Androgens, 119. *See also* Hormones
Anemia, 53
Anexsia 5/500, 235
Anexsia 7.5/650, 235
Anger, 83–84
Anodynos, 30–31
Ansaid, 100, 125, 132, 193. *See also* Flurbiprofen
Antacids, 75
Anticonvulsants, 11, 201
Antidepressants, 11; for adolescents' headaches, 182–83; for children's headaches, 178–79; headaches caused by, 202; influence on serotonin levels, 6; for migraines, 92–97; for post-

traumatic headaches, 192; side effects of, 96–97; for tension headaches, 129–31, 135
Antihistamines, in Norgesic Forte, 181
Anti-inflammatories. *See* Nonsteroidal anti-inflammatories (NSAIDs)
Antinausea medication, 151–52, 234
Anxiety, 5, 6, 7, 55, 83–84, 123, 191
Aphasia, 55
Aristocort, 153. *See also* Triamcinolone
Arrestin, 77. *See also* Trimethobenzamide
Arthritis, 53, 131, 177
Arthritis Strength BC Powder, 228
Arthritis Strength Bufferin Analgesic, 229
Ascriptin, Regular Strength and Extra Strength, 228
Ascriptin A/D, 228
Aspartame, 87
Aspirin: for adolescents' headaches, 180–81; for after-surgery headaches, 199; in Anacin, 33, 180; for children's headaches, 173–74; description of, 32; in Excedrin Extra-Strength, 30, 181; for hangovers, 198; headaches caused by, 202; in Norgesic Forte, 65, 126, 181; in over-the-counter pain relievers, 30; for post-traumatic headaches, 191; and rebound headaches, 7; as a self-help strategy, 19; side effects of, 32, 124; for tension headaches, 124, 133. *See also* Nonsteroidal anti-inflammatories (NSAIDs)
Aspirin Free Anacin, 225
Aspirin Free Anacin P.M., 225
Aspirin-Free Excedrin, 32, 63, 168–69, 180, 225. *See also* Nonsteroidal anti-inflammatories (NSAIDs)
Aspirin with codeine, 236
Association for Applied Psychophysiology and Feedback, 221
Asthma, 97, 98, 178
Atenolol, 98, 118, 201. *See also* Beta-blockers
Ativan, 235
Auras, 12, 55, 56, 57, 58
Autogenic training, 21, 24–25; exercise, 24–25
Aventyl: for adolescents' headaches, 182–83; for children's headaches,

Psychotherapy, 36–39, 84–85, 191, 213, 222–23
Pulsatilla, 210

Radiofrequency trigeminal rhizotomy, 159
Ranitidine, 201
Raynaud's syndrome, 97, 101
Rebound headaches: in adolescents, 182; from caffeine, 3, 7–8, 15, 29, 59, 125, 202; description of, 7–8; from ergotamines, 8, 155, 202; from ergotamine tartrate, 148–49; incidence of, 7, 8; from over-the-counter pain relievers, 7–8, 13, 30, 31, 53, 59, 124, 202; from sumatriptan, 68; as transformed migraines, 53
Record keeping, 47. See also Calendar, for headache tracking
Reglan, 64, 76, 107. See also Metoclopramide
Relafen, 132. See also Nonsteroidal anti-inflammatories (NSAIDs)
"Relaxation response," 21
Relaxation techniques, 4, 9, 17, 19–27, 59, 117, 122, 123, 167, 179, 191, 213
Remedies: failure to take advantage of, 2–3; home, 209; homeopathic, 205, 210–11
Reserpine, 36
Respiratory infections and illnesses, 19, 45, 53
Retrogasserian injection of glycerol, 159
Reye's syndrome, 172, 173
Ritalin, 107, 136. See also Methylphenidate
Robaxin, 134, 191. See also Methocarbamol
Robbins Headache Clinic, 137
Rolaids, 31, 75
Rufen, 31–32, 64, 125. See also Ibuprofen

S-A-C tablets, 30–31
St. Joseph Adult Chewable Aspirin, 228
St. Joseph Aspirin-Free Fever Reducer for Children, 226
Salatin, 30–31
Saleto, 30–31
Salt packs, 209
Sanguinaria, 210

Sansert, 103, 114, 154, 192. See also Methysergide
Seasons, 36, 83, 87–88
Sedatives, 72, 74, 127. See also Tranquilizers
Seizures, 19, 55, 204
Self-help strategies, 18–39, 213
Self-hypnosis, 25–26, 206; exercise, 26
Seligman, Dr. Martin E., 37
Serax, 237
Sergolexole maleate, 212
Serotonin, 5–7, 11, 13, 28, 59, 111, 123, 145
Sertraline, 95, 130. See also Antidepressants
Sex: as a headache remedy, 211; as a headache trigger, 15, 83, 89, 192–93
Sexuality, 191
Shingles, 201
Shower massager, 147
Side effects: of abortive medication, 9; of antidepressants, 96–97; of aspirin, 32; of migraines, 59, 75–77; of over-the-counter pain relievers, 30; of prescription medications, 3
Sinarest, 232
Sinarest Extra-Strength, 232
Sinarest No Drowsiness, 232
Sine-Aid Maximum Strength, 232
Sine-Off Maximum Strength No Drowsiness, 232
Sine-Off Sinus Medicine, Aspirin Formula, 233
Sinequan, 94, 131. See also Doxepin
Sinus disease, 45
Sinus Excedrin Analgesic Decongestant, 232
Sinus headaches, 12, 14, 195–96, 202
Sinus x-ray, 46
Sinutab Sinus Allergy Medication, 233
Sleep: excessive, 36, 83, 89; as headache relief, 122; lack of, 36, 54, 83, 88, 166; regular schedule of, 7, 214; and serotonin, 5. See also Insomnia
Smoke, 36, 54, 83, 88, 166, 196, 214
Smoking, 146
Sominex, 226
Sonazine, 77. See also Chlorpromazine
Sore throat, 19, 196